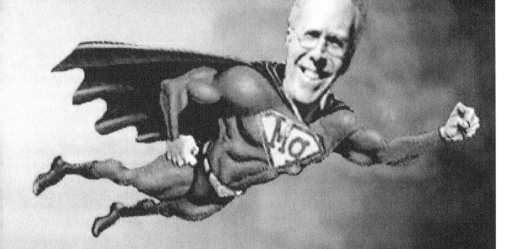

Musings From MAG...

volume two

Compiled By
Genelle Young

MAG**NESIUM**
ADVOCACY
GROUP

First edition, December, 2015
Volume II

Compiled by Genelle Young with permission of Morley Robbins

©2015, Genelle Young and Morley Robbins

Thank you to Michelle Stewart for Editing Support.
Thank you to Megan Young for Cover design, and Editing Support.

Disclaimer:

All information provided here out is completely general, and not specific to any one person. You need to know your mineral status, and have it interpreted by a trained interpreter to know which information would apply to you. Morley is happy to work with you to achieve optimum health via his website, for which a link is provided below. But, I am by no means qualified to do so and do not, at this current time, have the capacity to independently diagnose someone with any mineral deficiency. I am however willing to make suggestions based on my own knowledge.

All recommended supplements and products, at the time of this file being complied, was recommended to Morley and he advises the use of them based on research and information he has come across. He is in no way responsible for any unforeseen side-effects or issue that arise from the direct use of recommended products, nor am I. As companies develop their products, they may be altered in regards to their ingredients, so please check carefully and ask questions in regards to what you intend to take. You need to make sure you are getting what you need and that the supplements you are taking do not counteract each other.

Morley gets no throw back from these products in any way, so his opinion is not governed by any company and what is sold to you does not benefit him in any way. Please be advised that you should not avoid a proper consultation, do not self-diagnose or treat yourself based on the information provided to you, seek a professional opinion.

Morley encourages you to take responsibility for your own health care decisions based upon inspired research, and in partnership with a qualified health care professional who can think well outside the box of today's vogue, misguided, biologically-incorrect, but "politically-correct" medical and dietary recommendations that are fueling the epidemic of chronic disease worldwide.

Hi, my name is Genelle Young.

After following to Magnesium Advocacy Group for some time due to health issues, I decided to take the plunge and do the HTMA with Morley last January. It was such a relief for someone to put on paper that, "yes there is something out of balance". I had seen so many specialists and had so many tests over the years, a Diagnostic Physician even commented "You have been this way so long, so obviously you have learnt to live with it, it's not killing you, and what do you want me to do?"

I had tried endless alternative medicine and to be honest, when I looked into mineral balancing, I was not filled with confidence. And, not to mention, we all know the impact alternative choices can have on the old bank account. While I followed the wall, I would scroll in anticipation for Morley's replied and with great excitement, I would copy his notes. These notes grew and grew and grew. So, it was then that I started thinking that I could share these notes, knowing there had to be other people out there scrolling as I do, waiting for Morley's input, but felt it only right to ask Morley for his blessing. Morley's reply was, "Let's make this an Ebook". I was ecstatic, Morley Robbins wants to work with me?!

And so began the long hours of bringing this all together! I hope it just keeps getting bigger and bigger.

My husband (of 19 years) and I have 4 children, 2 girls, 2 boys, between 18 and 5. We also run our own self built retail business, which we have just expanded, and built a mechanic workshop onto. With so much spare time (can you hear my sarcasm here?), I thought, too easy! Not. (Does anyone else have any idea how much stuff Microsoft Word can do when you actually know how to use it?!) So, for me this has been a labor of love to assemble hoping that I can help people get a better understanding as to what the mineral balancing can do. I hope these notes I have complied, give you a better understanding that, No, you don't have to accept your aliments. Yes, there is help. I have entrusted Morley to Captain our journey's to better health and I have done HTMA's for all of my family, as we all have our quirks that I was looking to iron out. BUT, Mineral Balancing isn't a quick fix. It is a commitment of at least a year or two and most of all, a lifestyle change to maintain. It's not "let's do one HTMA and hope for the best" it is a long term dedication. But, I am sure when you get to the end of this book, you will be looking for that http://gotmag.org/ to get you started too.

I hope you enjoy the information, as much as I did compiling it!!!

Content

A Few Words About Magnesium Man

Morley M. Robbins

"There is no such thing as "medical disease..." There is only "metabolic dysfunction" that is CAUSED by "mineral deficiencies..."

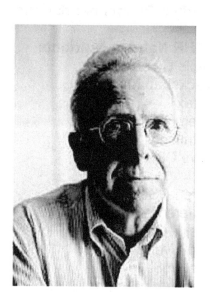

https://www.facebook.com/groups/MagnesiumAdvocacy/

http://gotmag.org/
morley@gotmag.com
847.922.8061

MAGNESIUM ADVOCACY GROUP Founder Morley M. Robbins (aka. "Magnesium Man") has a mainstream medical industry background. That's intriguing when you consider that he is now devoted to promoting natural and preventive health solutions.

Morley had been a hospital executive and consultant for 32 years when, several years ago, he developed a condition called "frozen shoulder." His family doctor quickly recommended surgery as the only hope for Morley if he wanted to be able to lift his right hand above his waist ever again.

Friends who owned a health food store intervened and encouraged Morley to try chiropractic care. His initial response:

 "Thanks guys, but I don't do witchcraft."

Several months later, the pain was wearing on him, and his friends insisted.

It only took a couple weeks of "light touch chiropractic care" (Network Spinal Analysis) before his shoulder had full range of motion once again.

The experience was so life-changing for Morley, he questioned everything he knew — or thought he knew — about healing.

He left the world of hospital administration and became a Wellness Coach.

Morley Discovers Mag

In July 2011, Morley was guided to read Carolyn Dean's wonderful book *The Magnesium Miracle*. He realized that nutrients, in general and magnesium, in particular, were a key piece of the whole health puzzle that virtually no practitioners seemed to be aware of — even in the natural health world.

He was captivated by this mineral, and went on to read even more. Much more...

Twenty-five books and 2500 articles (and counting) on mineral metabolism (ie Iron overload etc) Magnesium and Copper deficiency. Morley has come to realize that Magnesium and key minerals, plays a role in *all* key metabolic systems, and is therefore a contributing factor to nearly *all* major health issues.

Magnesium deficiency is the common thread for millions of Americans who are dealing with **heart disease, diabetes, obesity, osteoporosis, cancer, general fatigue, and any chronic condition borne out of inflammation**.

As Morley read and made connections between hundreds of scientific studies, what he found was shocking:

Magnesium deficiency, or insufficiency, was at the center of all these common modern diseases due to its central role in activating 3,751 proteins, and thus thousands of enzyme systems (far more than the Internet figure of 300 enzyme pathways...).

It became increasingly easy to see why this family of Magnesium-related health problems would be so common in modern life. Over the past century, drinking water treatment and food processing has removed naturally-occurring Magnesium from our dietary environment. Meanwhile stressful lifestyles cause our bodies to burn through what little Magnesium we do have inside us. Furthermore, many prescription medications are known to cause Magnesium, and other mineral loss, as well.

Morley has coined the phrase "Magnesium Burn Rate" (MBR) to help folks internalize the physical price they pay from the many "Stressors!" in their world.

Morley, in concert with his partner, "Dr. Liz" Erkenswick, DC, (who MAG-ically healed his shoulder…) began working with their clients on a program of natural healing, with particular emphasis on this "Magnesium deficiency issue."

Because of Magnesium, their clients' lives changed. Profoundly.

Their clients' "need" for statins, anti-depressants, digestive meds, sleeping pills, and osteoporosis medications (just to name a few) were effectively offset by concerted efforts to manage their stress response, eating REAL foods rich in minerals, vitamins and fats, and undertaking protocols to restore bio-available Magnesium supplements. (3 Steps to Restore Magnesium)

Morley had read the published studies on how Magnesium repletion could help reverse high cholesterol, cure low-grade depression, stop insomnia, increase bone density, and support hundreds of numerous other enzyme-dependent (and thus Magnesium-dependent) processes in the body…

But it was seeing the results in his clients' lives that really galvanized his purpose.

Today, Morley views it as his life's work to push back the tides of nutritional insanity and Magnesium deficiency in the day-to-day lives of inhabitants of Planet Earth!

Through MAG, he is committed to educating as many people as possible about the *MAG-nificence of Magnesium* and ending the epidemic of Magnesium deficiency plaguing the health and well-being of American society. Please join him in his Facebook, Magnesium Advocacy Group, to gain greater insights into the importance of minerals, in general, and Magnesium, in particular:

https://www.facebook.com/groups/MagnesiumAdvocacy/

Training

Morley did his primary HTMA training with Rick Malter, PhD, http://www.malterinstitute.org/ He has been guided by a dozen other gifted mineral reasearchers & experts, however.

~ A WORD FROM THE MAN HIMSELF ~

It's a bit more complicated than just one program and mentorship, although Rick Malter, PhD has been legendary:

o   I'm a Scorpio -- I LOVE to dig... .

o   I'm a contrarian -- I delight in challenging authority for sport...

o   I'm a conspiracist -- turns out it's NOT a conspiracy...

o   I failed miserably in college to study "science" so I could be a "doctor" -- got "No thanks!" from 18 schools... Ouch! (*And thank God for that!...*)

o   Discovered I had a gift for pattern recognition... Studied General Systems Theory in B-School and loved it!

o   Completed Reed Davis' FDN Program– highly recommend it!

o   Completed 2 of 3 levels of Freddie Ulan, DC's program Nutritional Response Testing -- MIND-BLOWING program...

o   Attended several seminars with Stuart White, DC -- a profoundly gifted practitioner, healer and educator...

o I was blessed to connect with my now wife, Dr. Liz, who is also a most gifted healer who taught me what natural healing is ALL about -- awakening the innate wisdom of the individual...

o Read Carolyn Dean, MD, ND's book, "The Magnesium Miracle," that changed my life... (Mostly for the better...)

o Went on to read 25 books or more and 2500 articles... and is still digging!...

o Completed the Institute for Integrated Nutrition Program...it's a wonderful program as it exposes you to 50+ different approaches to nutrition... it is, however, a "mineral desert" when it comes to training...

o I would be remiss to not mention my buddy, Peter Wisniewski (founder of http://endobalance.com/) who was the ONE who actually suggested I get into HTMA analysis, and then withstood months (years) of my "bitching" about how hard it was to understand and master... He also has been instrumental in teaching Dr. Liz and me about the amazing gifts of Standard Process supplements, that are magically designed for natural healing...

o It was because of Pete's suggestion that I took Rick Malter's course which I HIGHLY recommend to anyone seeking to practice HTMA analysis...

   I have had the added blessing of forging a friendship since 2009 with Rick that has shaped my thinking as a practitioner, but more importantly, as an awaking participant on this Planet!...

o   And last, but not least, was the two years I spent interacting with Patrick Sullivan Jr. during my time being sponsored by Jigsaw Health (2011-2013). Patrick is simply a class act (by the way, apples don't fall far from trees...) and he "created" the persona of "Magnesium Man!," fostered my confidence as a writer and speaker, and engaged in countless hours of dialogue about how best to communicate the gift of minerals, in general, and Maggie, in particular...

That ^^^^ is the looooong and short of my "training" as it were...

I'm confident that I'll start a "school" but the question is when... Likely in 2016 or 2017. Thank you all for taking an interest...

Hi From Morley

I am most OPEN to learning how to better use these diagnostic tools and welcome the input of other practitioners to learn from. As I've stated repeatedly, I don't pretend to have all the answers -- hardly.

What I do know, however, is that there's a great deal of confusion in conventional circles, in large part due to a failure to understand and incorporate mineral metabolism into the dynamics of metabolic dysfunction…

I have spent 32+ years as an executive in the health care field...

I made a very conscious choice in 2009 to step off the Allopathic grid and enlighten souls about how their bodies REALLY work, not how BIG Pharma and their Minion Deities want them to believe it works...

Please know, I don't pretend to have all the answers... Truly I don't. I do, however, have a very different perspective on human metabolisum, based on the mineral functions that run the body.

What I can say is that I have NO fear of standing with an umbrella in the face of a TIDAL WAVE of "D"isinformation and "D"eception that floods MOST conventional articles and research on health, nutrition and healing.

We have been Misled... We have been Misfed... Truth be known, we have "Missing Minerals" -- mostly!

I have recognised degrees:

o   "PhD", which stands for "Passionate hatred for Disinformation"... And an

o   "MD", which stands for "Mineral Detective"

Each of which are "Honorary" and bestowed to me by the Wizard of Oz!

MAG is littered with hundreds (thousands?...) of folks who have been abused by an insensitive, arrogant, and in my humble opinion, under-trained medical system devoid of common sense or willingness to sort out the metabolic foundation revealed by minerals...

There are hundreds of folks who requested the Mag RBC only to get a serum Mg which is entirely worthless as a diagnostic tool. Yet doctors contiuly order serum Mg, largely due to their limited training.

As for the cost, it can be expensive, but there, too, many, many folks have WASTED thousands of $$£££€€¥¥ in the vortex of conventional medicine...

Trust me, I hear upward of twenty five stories per week -- each one more heart-breaking than the last... The level of clinical incompetence is mind-numbing, quite frankly.

So, my sincere recommendation to ALL, is to take action -- outside the BOX of convention -- and take control of your health and steps to bring your body back into balance.

And in closing, I would encourage all to STOP "hoping and praying" that your doctor will finally figure this out... Their training is designed to treat disease - NOT cure it. There are many theories on "WHY" this is the case. All are speculative. The bottom line is that they are NOT trained in minerals, NOR mineral metabolism. Period.

Conventinal practitioners are not exactly flocking to my Facebook page -- nor am I expecting them to -- and nor should you, either...

I am growing weary of "labels" that the average person fears and the average practitioner does NOT understand, metabolically.

100% of the people on the MAG group are "Stress! Cadets" and thus mineral deserts... from 3-4 generations of overly processed folks, as well as abject denial re the vital importance of minerals to run the body.

Welcome to new MAG members.

Here's the link to Mildred S. Seelig, MD, MPH Magnus Opus: Re the fundemental ESSENTIALITY of MAG in our lives -

http://www.mgwater.com/.../Magnesium.../preface.shtml

That will keep you occupied for a couple of weeks, at least...

And please know we've never met a question we didn't enjoy!

Affiliated Practitioners

HTMA Practitioners affiliated with the Magnesium Advocacy Group

Morley Robbins, CHC

Rick Malter, PhD

Robert Thompson, MD

Julie Casper, LAc

Pippa Galea

Wendy Myers

Eileen Durphy

Dede Moore – EFT Practitioner

EFT aka Emotional Freedom Technique is acupuncture without the needles, with an added emotional component. We cannot separate body from mind. This is an easy and amazing tool to boost and promote your overall heath, as well as eradicate issues that you think are only physical.

A couple of reasons to use EFT:

1) It is an easy and effective way to handle stress and reduce our MBR.

2) If you have tried several things to physically feel better, and they're not working.

3) You consider your past or your present full of "Stressful!" or emotional situations.

A couple of reasons to work with a certified EFT Practitioner:

1) They are trained to see what you can't see. For example, you might think you need to work on your marriage when really there is an issue from your childhood.

2) In EFT lingo, you are borrowing the benefits which means you actually benefit from the energy of the trained Practitioner.

3) If you want to get to the Olympics competing as a runner you wouldn't just run, you would get a trainer.

4) People drawn to this issue of minerals and mineral deficiency tend to be smart. Smart people like to be in control. For EFT to work it's MAG-ic, we need to "surrender". That is best achieved when working with a practitioner trained in the process.

Members of the MAG group are fortunate enough to have a very gifted EFT Practitioner among us! Dede Moore generously offers the first session free. You can contact Dede at eft4anxiety@gmail.com

I took Dede up on her standing offer to the MAG-pie community: One free EFT session to try it. I have been doing weekly sessions for the past 4-5 months and was blown away by what it has done for me. Dede is incredibly gifted in her skills, she has applied this AMAZING EFT tool to a number of key issues, (aka, emotional knots) and they are GONE!...

I am very grateful that our paths crossed and that she is so talented at what she does. I would encourage you and any others, who are dealing with emotional issues at the core of their mineral imbalances – which would be 100% of us!!!

Again, enviromental stress is very often the origin of our MBR.

MINERALS

Magnesium: A Beginners Guide To Mag

Even though roughly over 80+% of the population is Mg deficient, we still recommend testing first.

http://gotmag.org/magnesium-deficiency-101/

Mg RBC (Functional range is 5.0-7.0 mg/dL, strive for 6.5! But 7.0 is heaven.)

Blood Test

http://requestatest.com/magnesium-rbc-testing

Hair Tissue Mineral Analysis

http://gotmag.org/work-with-us/

How to Restore Magnesium

http://gotmag.org/how-to-restore-magnesium/

Critical co-factors for Mg absorption:

B6 helps get Magnesium INSIDE the cell (recommended brand's are Jigsaw Health Mg SRT and MagKey as they contains B6, Mg co-factor.)

Boron helps KEEP mag INSIDE the cell (Anderson's Concentrated Minerals or Aussie Sea Minerals, Relyte, as well as prunes and raisins, that contain much needed trace mineral, boron.)

Sodium Bicarbonate helps get Mag Inside the Mitochondria. (Mag water)

Selenium and Taurine and are added co-factors to improve Mg intake and retention...

Where Mg is found in our body:

SAVINGS o 60% in bones.

CHECKING o 27% in muscle with the highest concentration in the ventricles of the heart.

DEBIT o 12% in soft tissue (heart, brain, liver, kidney, endocrine glands and related tissues)

WALLET o 1% in the blood it comes out of "storage" in tissue and components of the blood 1st, bones 2nd, and lastly from serum which is why Mg serum tests are worthless.

Magnesium: How To Restore Mag

I am often asked, "So how much Magnesium do I need to take daily?"

It's a great question. And like most great questions, the answer is, "It depends."

There are actually 3 points to consider:

1) Increased S*T*R*E*S*S = Increased MBR

First, please know that stress consumes Magnesium (Mg) — it's how we're wired as a species. The more "Stress!" you are under, the more Magnesium your body burns. Please take a moment to re-read that...

I call this the "Magnesium Burn Rate", or MBR. It's the metabolic price we pay for all that pressure, tension and change we all feel.

Take an inventory of the dimensions of stress... Food allergies, dependence on processed food, exposure to heavy metals, use of Rx drugs, and the granddaddy of them all — mental and emotional stress, to name but a few of the "Stressors" that deplete our Mg stores. Take whatever steps you can to mitigate these issues to shore up these Mg leaks.

And when you know your "Stress!"/MBR is increasing, know that your body will be craving more Magnesium.

2) What is your Current Magnesium Status?

The most efficient and cost-effective way to get a reading on your current Magnesium status is to order the MagRBC blood test (available from Request a Test).

This simple test costs $49 and you'll usually have results emailed to you within 72 hours, for those who reside in the states.

The current Lab reference range is 4.2 – 6.8 mg/dL, but know that in 1962 (before every 1/3 person was obese, diabetic or addicted to RX meds) the Reference Range was 5.0-7.0mg/dL (**/2.43 for mmol/L). Based on this latter Range, any score below 6.0 mg/dL is a clear signal of Magnesium deficiency. Ideally, we **STRIVE** to get the Mag RBC to **6.5**, 7 is Heaven!

If you have many Magnesium deficiency symptoms (http://gotmag.org/magnesium-deficiency-101/), an even less expensive option is to just start increasing your Magnesium intake. See the next step…

3) Protocol for Restoring Magnesium

- **Diet** – Start eating more Magnesium-rich foods: Seafood, especially kelp and oysters. Whole grains, especially buckwheat, millet and wild rice. Leafy greens, especially Collards, Beet Greens, Mustard Greens, spinach and kale. Nuts and seeds, especially cashews, almonds, and pistachio nuts, as well as pumpkin seeds.

And everyone's favorite, Chocolate! But, only dark chocolate with a high content of Cacao, 80% or more is best!

(NOTE: Because of mineral depletion in the soil and modern food processing methods, I've determined that it's basically impossible to get enough Magnesium from food alone, so please continue reading…)

- **Magnesium Mineral Drops** – Put Anderson's Concentrated Mineral, or Aussie Sea Minerals or Relyte, drops in your water — minerals are the *other* "element" we're looking for when we are thirsty for H2O!

- **Magnesium Oil Footbath's** – Do a magnesium oil footbath. If you can't do it daily, at least 2-3X/week to replenish extreme magnesium deficiency rapidly. Dose is 1 – 2 oz of Magnesium Oil plus ½ cup of baking soda and ½ tbsp of borax in enough hot water to cover your toes in a small tub.

- **Epsom Salt/Mg Chloride Flakes Bath** – Magnesium baths are great. Grandma used to recommend them for just about everything! And Epsom Salt (Magnesium Sulfate) is readily available at just about every local drugstore, and Mg Cl flakes at your local health food store. Dose is 1-2 cups of Epsom Salt or Mg Cl flakes (NEVER TOGETHER) + 1 Cup of Baking Soda (*not* baking powder) plus 1 Tbsp of Borax, and immerse yourself in this rejuvenating liquid for 30-40 min. I recommend slowing down and enjoying one per week.

Please know Mg Chloride oil out performs Epsom Salt if the objective is to increase Mg levels... Epsom salt, however is superior for detox... I've studied this carefully with clients and those with the fastest rise in Mg status all make liberal use of Mg Chloride oil, either through baths or transdermal spray.

But if "slowing down" isn't in your vocabulary, continue reading…

- **Magnesium Supplements** – Take a bio-available Magnesium supplement *every* day.

Three brands that I confidently recommend are Jigsaw Magnesium withSRT (time release), Magnesium Glycinate by Pure Encapsulations, MagKey.

(NOTE: No matter what magnesium supplement you use, be sure to also supplement with vitamin B6, an important co-factor to Magnesium absorption. To this point, I give a slight edge to <u>Jigsaw</u> and <u>MagKey</u> since their formulas already include B6.)

The Recommended Daily Intake (RDI) of Magnesium is 400mg. But I believe the Optimal Daily Dose is 650mg for Women and 850mg for men, but please vary it based upon your daily Magnesium Burn Rate.

My preferred rule of thumb is to take 5mg/lb or 10mg/kg your body weight in mgs of Mg (e.g. If you weigh 100 lbs / or 50 kilos, take 500 mgs Mg.) That is to maintain your Mg status, take more to restore, or adress your increased MBR.

Again, the focus here is on "optimum" dosing, not daily "minimum" intakes.

4) One Last Thing…

OK, now this last part is quite difficult, so please pay close attention…

I'd like you to do this degree of Mg supplementation each and every day. We have THREE key daily absolutes:

Air, Water, Magnesium — it's that important!

And when you start increasing your Magnesium intake, you'll be fueling your body with *the* Master Mineral that powers *all* 100 Trillion cells, especially the largest muscle in your body, your non-stop beating heart.

Magnesium: What's Your Mag Status

Please know that the MAG functional Range for optimal Health is 5.0-7.0mg/dL. 6.5 is optimal, 7 is heaven. [**mg/dl / 2.43**= mmol/L] (The current lab range is based on very chronically ill people...)

When Mg is deficient, here's what's impacted:

o   Autonomic Nervous System gets agitated, our response to "Stress!" Gets our system agrivated.

o   Energy production (ATP Production) gets affected.

o   3,751 proteins are affected, especailly in the mitachondria.

o   Iron absorption and transport is affected which lead to Anemia...

o   B12 can't get INSIDE the cell (the enzyme is dependent on Mg-ATP!), and builds up in the blood...

Suggestion, do your best to bypass the Xanax as it will only further deplete your Mg, Cu, Zn and Fe, work on restoring your Mg status

www.gotmag.org/how-to-restore-magnesium/

Pursue multiple channels of Mg recovery... BEFORE you resort to shots, etc.

Magnesium: Deficiency Symptoms

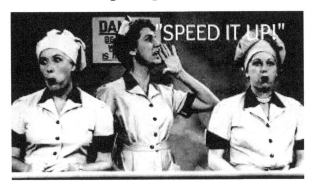

What causes MAG loss....

Physical, Metabolic, Emotional, Environmental, and Nutritional "Stressors!"

Among the MOST damaging sources of Mg Loss:

o   Exposure to Fluoride...
o   Anesthesia...
o   Rx medications...
o   Emotional Shock (death of a loved one, etc.)
o   Car Accidents
o   Iron Overload

These are some good sources for you...

http://bja.oxfordjournals.org/content/83/2/302.full.pdf

http://ckj.oxfordjournals.org/content/5/Suppl_1.toc

http://www.mgwater.com/.../Magnesium.../Preface.shtml

http://www.lef.org/.../may2008_Magnesium-Widespread...

http://www.mgwater.com/rodtitle.shtml

That ought to keep you in the Library for at least a couple of hours... There's plenty more where those came from...

As a former "hospital jockey," I had NO idea how CENTRAL Magnesium was to optimal health or how its deficiency was the CAUSE to most, if not ALL, chronic disease.

Picture a "hub and spoke" wheel. At the core is Mg deficiency, and the spokes are the hundreds/thousands of enzyme pathways --that are Mag dependent-- that when they stop firing, CAUSE the conditions that we have been "trained" to believe is "disease." They are NOT disease. They are nutritional deficiencies, that menifest as symptoms and pain

Even "auto-immune" conditions...

http://www.rense.com/general83/fount.htm

http://www.nutritionalmagnesium.org/magnesium-deficiency.../

The resilience of the human body exceeds anything I know of... Remove the "Stressors!" and feed the body balanced nutrients, and my reading of the literature suggests that virtually all conditions are reversible...

For those that will come down hard on me for saying that, it just may be that we have NOT learned how to do the above in all its forms...

Part of the challenge in our health recovery, is our limited belief in the "lack of reversibility," or the "lack of resilience" of the human metabolism.

Magnesium: Mag Your Bath

Epsom Salt is more of a detox...

Mg Chloride flakes is more of a source for Mg restoration...
Mg Cl flakes are uses to make Mg Cl oil or to place in a tub for a bath... it's more long-term recovery...

Epsom salts (Mg SO4) is another form of Mg that is used for bathing... its more short-term relief

Baking Soda (Sodium Bicarbonate) is added to water to make it more Alkaline... It does NOT contain Borax... You can use up to 2 Cup/bath...

Borax (Boron) is a mineral with known properties to help regulate the Calcium/Magnesium dance... Yes the washing power!!! 1 tbsp is a good dose for each full bath, or 1/2 tbsp for each foot bath.

Magnesium: Milk Of Magnesia

MoM (aka, Mg hydroxide, Mg (on)z) was invented in 1873 and has been used throughout the world for ~150 years... It has known properties for both antiacid and laxative....Why is it being banned in Europe, U.K. and Down Under?!?

BECAUSE IT WORKS!!!

All is NOT as it seems...

Please read this slooooowly:

http://monthlyaspectarian.com/morley-August-2012.html

I can properly speak far more eloquently to the efforts underway around the Globe to restrict access to minerals and supplements to the non-Priestly group of citizens that make up the 99.9% of the population.

It is a dark, dark chapter in the evolution of the world...

That said, I have NO insider information on why this is happening. What I have noted is that the following Mg-based products are more, and more impossible to find:

o   Carter's Liver pills...
o   Doan's Back pills...
o   Bufferin (Aspirin buffered with Mg!)
o   and numerous others...

And what are these being replaced with? NSAIDS!

And what's a distinctive feature of NSAIDs?

They create Magnesium loss, and devastate the production of Glutathime.

Hmmmmm... Think that's a coincidence?... Nope, me neither!

Please note Bullet #3 in the attached article:

http://www.askdrmaxwell.com/.../do-you-have-a-magnesium.../

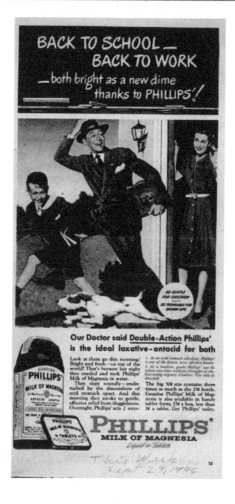

34

MOTHER WAS RIGHT: THE HEALTH BENEFITS OF MILK OF MAGNESIA

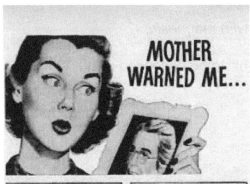

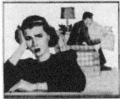
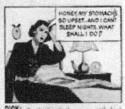
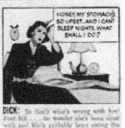
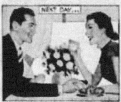

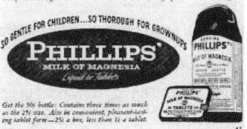

MAG-pies of the "Mother" Persuasion -- Alert!
May one and ALL of the Moms that grace this MOM-crazed group have a blessed and wonderful Day! And as a MAG-appropriate present, I present to you the wonderful writing of Marshall Alan Wolf, MD, one of the greatest Cardiologists to train future such doctors at Harvard's Brigham and Women's Hospital...

http://www.ncbi.nlm.nih.gov/.../PMC150.../pdf/tacca117000001.pdf

(I was absolutely humbled and honored to chat with him a couple of years ago to thank him for and to discuss this delightful article...)
May you find comfort and wisdom in his observations about BOTH his Mom, and Maggie!...

Magnesium: Morley's Mag Obsession

Is it "healthy" to be obsessed with magnesium?

As a nation, we've been "taught" to be obsessed with:

o   Calcium...
o   Cholesterol...
o   "Low Fat!"...
o   Tons of "D!"...
o   No Salt!...
o   No Red Meat...
o   No Eggs!...
o   and on, and on, and on, and on...

All of which has been proven to be pure poppycock! (Yes, even the vaulted "D"ietary "D"ictum on "D" is "D"ying... Thank God!)

At least by focusing on Maggie, we're restoring the metabolic foundation of the human body to resume its natural role in quietly regulating and balancing and energizing thousands upon thousands of functions that allow us to be symptom-free and Rx med-free!

In my humble opinion, it beats our earlier programming by factors thousands-fold...

Truly, why are people wasting their time trying to "convince" their doctor regarding a Mg blood test?!?

What was most telling in that exchange: "If Mg were important they would test for it."

The FACT that the doctor does NOT test for it SAYS IT ALL FOLKS!...

It's not just "important," -- it's CENTRAL to understanding the metabolic health of the individual...And the fact that you've never heard that before does NOT mean it's wrong.

Sheeeeseeesh...

When was the last time you updated your understanding of the extensive network of metabolic, detox and energy pathways that are ENTIRELY dependent on Mg status?...

There are countless secondary and tertiary pathways that begin to malfunction when the cell, and key enzyme pathways, are no longer able to produce energy (Mg-ATP) efficiently...
If you are relying on the filtered textbook(s) of Physiology that you studied in Medical School, your knowledge base is seriously flawed... more like "Swiss Cheese," than based on definitive science...

I don't take lightly to "practitioners" who received their education from BIG Pharma-funded schools of Rx dispensing acting as "experts" on "disease" when they have flawed education, the mineral-depandant metabolic pathway that runs our body and our innate healing abilities.

Be ready for significant and scientific pushback on my end with a clear intent of informing the masses that when ALL THE DUST settles, the ultimate hinge for disease and dysfunction is a "LACK

OF ENERGY" (Mg-ATP) that is largely a Mg status issue --
induced by a wide spectrum of "Stressors!" -- just as Karl Fiedler
MD theorized in 1899, and his protégé, Hans Selye, MD, PhD,
ScD was able to prove in the 30,000 experiments that he
conducted with all manner of species during his illustrious and
storied 50-yr career, defining and codifying The General
Adaptatin Syndrome (GAS) that is the intellectual bedrock of
"Stress!" and it's impact on our physiology and immune systems.

Magnesium: Reactions

There are ~25 different forms of Maggie... I know not why, but we all do not respond well to different forms...

Hang in there and see how you respond to other forms...

In chatting with a noted pathologist about the "accuracy" of the Mag RBC test, he pointed out that the error can be up to +/- 20%, which is a significant # when you think about it...

Point.... Counter Point...

o   Mg Malate and Mg Glycinate are among the MOST effective in their absorption and impact... These are our "go to" oral Mg supplements...

o   Mg Cl oil -- transdermal -- has been used successfully for thousands of generations by folks who live near the Sea...

o   Mg Taurate is a wonderful form that is especially effective for those dealing with Heart muscle issues...

o   Mg Citrate is well absorbed, but MANY are affected by the fact that the Citrate molecule irritates the intestinal lining... Moving waste via "irritation" is NOT the same as metabolic "stimulation..."

o   Epsom salt (Mg Sulfate) has been used effectively since the LATE 1500's as a powerful detox and relaxing agent...

o   Mg Hydroxide (MoM) is MOST effective -- when used
     properly. Its use and effectiveness since its discovery in
     the late 1800's is legendary... MJ Hamp has a proven use
     for making Mg water that has helped MANY MAG-pies on
     this FB Group...

o   Mg Threonate is the latest, but NOT the only Mg to
     cross the BBB. It IS the form that has the BEST PR
     campaign that is designed to convince you that
     "Patented" Minerals is the way to go! (You should be
     VERY worried about THAT aspect of this product...)

Albion Minerals is the source for Jigsaw's Mg SRT and the two
forms of Mg Glycinate that we use, in our wellness center in
Louisiana: Doctor's Best, and PURE Encapsulations...

Keep in mind, Jigsaw INCLUDES the needed B's (And YES, the
Folate is the RIGHT kind...) and the Mg Glycinate requires the
addition of the B6, etc.

Remember Magnesium's role in the body is to regulate levels of
thousands of proteins that then affects minerals, vitamins,
enzymes, hormones, neurotransmitters, and genes...

Maggie is powerful mineral that plays a key role in many, many,
many activities.

It's important to know that Cortisol is your friend and when it's
low, it's likely that you've got too little Potassium, brought on by
Adrenal Fatigue that becomes Adrenal Suppression that causes
a systemic loss of Sodium and Potassium. And excess Calcium,

bio-unavailable Copper and Hormone-D work wonders to keep the Potassium in a state of deficiency...

It's a very dynamic process, and while hard to believe, is kept in balance and in motion when the body is allowed to keep its Magnesium status at optimal levels... It truly is the "Conductor of the Cell's Orchestra of Minerals..."

If you get lighted headed when starting Mag:

o   It's important to understand that the Adrenals are RULED by the mineral ratio of Sodium/Magnesium (Na/Mg)

o   Very likely, your Adrenals are whipped, which means that your Sodium (Na) is on the LOW side...

o   Infusion of Mg causes the Na/Mg ratio to get more inverted, this slooows your down more.

o   Very likely, you need Adrenal support to elevate your Sodium as the "light headed" feeling is associated with low Sodium which then affects fluid volume...

I would advise three things:

1)   Get a broad based assessment of your minerals, via an HTMA

2)   Read and act on this:
      http://gotmag.org/how-to-restore-magnesium/

3) Take the Adrenal Cocktail to support your body's need for minerals to feed the Adrenals…

Knowing you're "whipped," that's what I'd do… take several days (up to 2 weeks) to nourish the Adrenals with the minerals they've been missing and then start up the Maggie, again, but do so slooooooowly…

Getting tired following an infusion of Maggie is either a possible Detox reaction (pathways get fired up when Mg-ATP is around…) or it is a sign of weak Adrenals, given that these "Stress!" Glands are ruled by the mineral ratio of Sodium/Mg. So, when you pump in a lot of Mg, without mineral and vitamin support for the Adrenals, (seperate Na and wholefood Vit-C) the ratio goes south and so, too, does your energy level.

The unintended backside to "Mo' Maggie" is that it can cause an inversion in the Adrenal Ratio (Na/Mg). The BIGGER the Mg, the more it can drive the Adrenal Ratio South which will cause you to feel "exhausted!" I wonder if that might not be part of your dynamic…

You might want to try Adrenal Cocktail and see how you respond to some targeted Adrenal support...

One way you can test whether this latter issue is the cause is to try the Adrenal Cocktail 2-3 times and see how you respond to an infusion of targeted minerals (Sea Salt and Potassium [Cream of Tartar])

1/4 tsp Sea Salt
1/4 tsp Cream of Tartar (Potassium)
1/2 cup of Fresh squeezed Orange or Lime Juice (NOT Store

bought!...)

Drink at 10am and/or 3pm and see how you feel for several days...

80% of folks who try this, feel energized by this, the other 20% -- not so much. And thats o.k, there are other options, but this is the most fundemental approach.

Ultimately, you'll need focused nutritional support for your Adrenals, assuming that this is a key factor (which I suspect it is...), but this will give you support in the interim...

Just like adding oil to your car engine, it's always best to check the "dipstick" to find out how low you REALLY are... and this is true of people and minerals, too...

Best way to assess this is via an HTMA... This is discussed here:

www.gotmag.org/work-with-us/

Totally agree that "Adrenal Support" is needed in addition to the Adrenal Cocktail. At the end of the day, these "Stress!" Glands need to be re-built, and re-energise... which is accelerated with the use of herbal adaptogens, like Ashwaganda, Rhodiola, Licorice Root, holy basil, etc...

These approaches are very potent and need to be administered with direction of a practitioner, and in proper context that comes from mineral testing (HTMA, etc.)

Mg causes most to relax, but excites others... I wish I knew why...

The reasons for "agitated" sleep are likely:

o   Excess Calcium (it is the mineral that keeps you in
     Sympathetic Dominance..."Fight or flight"...)

o   Too little Potassium, as it is the mineral that enables the
     Parasympethetic response -- "Rest and recovery"

o   Excess, unbound Copper/ and or Iron (keeps you in
     HYPER-Sympathetic Dominance! And they disrupts the
     Melatonin Pathway -- badly!)

o   Too little Sodium (Electrolyte Derangement is very
     disruptive...)

What keeps these three issues in proper alignment? Optimal Mg
status, but without knowing your "mineral wiring" you will be
engaged in the "Bill Murray 'Caddyshack' Strategy of
Supplementation..."

A foundational starting point is testing and assessing your
mineral profile -- not just blindly throwing the latest vitamin or
neurotransmitter -- (both of which serve at the pleasure of the
minerals) into your metabolism.

You can be "neurologically switched," which is not uncommon
these days with the food additives and environmental toxins.
Don't mean to play a wild card here, but folks who have a
"HYPER" response to Maggie, need to be sensitive to taking it in
the am and may need to assess what other factors may be at
play, in this atypical response.

Please know that each member of the MAG Community has a different biochemical make-up. The fact that one person has a reaction, means that that person has had a reaction and should NOT become a basis of decision-making on your part.

The key here is to understand that Mineral restoration, with a particular emphasis on Maggie, is the key strategy for our metabolic function and dis-ease elimination. What is important is for you to experiment with different forms of Mg and determine what works in YOUR body...

Again, this is explained here:
www.gotmag.org/how-to-restore-magnesium/

Please take the time to engage in testing to have a proper mineral context for the efforts that you'll undertake with your diet and nutrition...

It is a very rare thing for Americans to be able to eat enough Magnesium in the typical, processed Diet.

Rare?...

It's more like, "next to impossible!"

Why's that?

o   Fluoride everywhere...

o   Excess dietary and supplement of Calcium and Iron...

o   Excess Hormone-D-- that is "Calcium on Steroids!"

o   Commercial agriculture that is an abomination to
       food, due to fertalizers and herbicides, etc...

o   Toxic industrial oils, like soybean, canolam corn oil, etc...

o   Excess dependence on Magnesuric Rx meds... (that
       means they CAUSE Mg to exit via the urine)

o   Excess Sugars and HFCS...

o   Excess MSG...(destroys glutamate, that burns up
       minerals)

o   Relentless "Stressors!" that constantly deplete minerals...

And this ^^^^ is just the headlines...

I know that you know this... this is just re-inforces for the MAG-
pies!

And, remember those Co-Factors---

These "status quo" RBC results are confounding... Me thinks it is
multiple factors that need to be accounted for and addressed:

What is the status of:

o   Plasma Zinc

o   Serum Copper

o   B6 intake

o   Boron

o   Bicarbonate

o   Taurate status (that affects B6)

o   Excess, unbound Copper status (that kills Mg, B6 and Zinc!)

o   Excess unbound Iron status (that kills Mg, B6 and Zinc)

o   Selenium status, needed for glutathione.

o   pH of the body, which is noteably affected by "Stressors!"

o   Effect of "Stressors!" not accounted for... [i.e. Mg Blocking Factors (Rx meds, excess Calcium, excess sugars, excess Hormone-D, etc.]

It's unusual to be taking this much Mg and feel no benefit. It suggests the Mg is NOT getting inside the cell.

o   The cofactors (noted previuosly) get Mg into cell

o   Boron helps keep it in the cell

o   Copper, and/or Iron, has a decided effect on Zinc, B6, and Mg. If the either levels are out of control, it is likely the Mg uptake will be challenged. Happy to discuss this further as you have the time and/or interest...

This process of restoring Mg status is VERY MUCH a Debits and Credits phenomenon... It is NOT just about taking Mo' Maggie!

It IS about managing the MBR (Mg Burn Rate)... And making sure we are accounting for the Mg leaks as well as the Mg intake -- properly supported with co-factors to get and keep the Mg INSIDE the cells...

Are you feeling better and are your symptoms melting away?!?... Not an insignificant component that deserves serious consideration...

At the end of the day, I want the MAG-pies to know that the forms of Mg therapy are rich and diverse...

There are compelling success stories whether we are talking about Mg MSM, Chelated Mg, Epsom Salts, Mg drops for water, Mg Bicarbonate, Mg-rich foods...

At first, it will appear a bit overwhelming... but as you become better versed in the MAG-ic of Magnesium, you will find that there are forms that you respond best to. And ideally, you will find 2-3 different forms so as to provide a bit of diversity for your bored little body that has been deprived of this mineral for faaaaar too long.

Don't hesitate to ask questions -- it's why we're here. We want a significant portion of the Planet to discover the role that this foundational mineral plays and that there are numerous ways to bring Maggie back to our cells. All forms are welcomed!

Two industries were born from global Magnesium deficiency:

o   Allopathic pharmaceutical industry...(which is largely composed of synthetic chemicals doing the job of Magnesium when it is insufficient inside the human body...)

o   Alternative supplement industry... (Which is largely composed of synthetic-derived supplements made by the very same companies in the 1st bullet point...)

Glycinate can be overstimulating...

I would first encourage you to get a Mag RBC to understand the metabolic origin of your symptoms and feelings of "Stress!"

Other options: Mg Cl Oil, Mg Water, and/or Mg Malate (Jigsaw), Mg Taurate, or Mg Orotate are proven to absorb well. Mg L-Threonate is another viable option.

o   Please note the Nutrition Therapy of this overview of Mitral Valve Prolapse (MVP) by Dr. Hoffman:

http://drhoffman.com/article/mitral-valve-prolapse-3/

Copper: Factors To Consider

To assess Copper Toxicity via blood, you must do four tests:

o   Mag RBC

o   Serum Copper

o   Serum Ceruloplasmin (Cp)

o   Plasma Zinc

There are two formulas to then assess the status (I.e. the level of unbound) Copper...Serum Copper - (3XCp) = "Free Cu"

Copper is very complicated. But this website answers most questions:

http://skinbiology.com/copper-the-protective-antiaging-meta

Loren Pickart, PhD is a genius, deserves a Nobel, but will byt the way NEVER get it...WHY?!? He pulled back the curtain to reveal just how VITAL and CENTRAL Copper is to our well-being...

I am more incline to simplify this process, and determine the level of "USABLE" Copper, which is simply serum Cp x3 = the amount of Copper that is bioavailable.

That is "excess, unbound Copper." Its removal requires strengthening the Adrenals and providing targeted nutrients to release the Copper:

o   Whole Vit-C Complex (NOT Ascorbic Acid!)

o   Broad-based B-Vitamins (especially B6)

o   Broad-based min (and Mg!)

o   Binding agent (Black Radish)

o   Liver support

This is best done under the direction of a practitioner who understands the metabolic processes involved, in restoring Copper metabolisum NOT seeking to "DETOX" it's removal!

HTMA is absolutely enough, but the Western world has been conditioned to believe that "blood is best" -- when, in fact, it is widely misused and grossly misinterpreted.

So, I use "blood" to appeal to people's subconscious programming, which is very deep... It's an increased expense, but it works, the interplay of the HTMA and blood tests is very powerful...

As for terminology, "Copper Toxicity" is a double-entendre: -- it means TWO states that co-exist;

o   Excess, unbound Copper, AND
o   Too little bio-available Copper

They are flipsides of the same coin.
And HOW does this happen?!?

When your Adrenals get "fried" from excess "Stressors!" (and too little mineral support, ahem!...), they are unable to:

1)   Signal the need to produce Ceruloplasmin (Cp) in the Liver, which needed to bind to the influx of Copper... and

2)   Produce adequate Mg-ATP to bind Copper to its target protein, Ceruloplasmin, which requires that molecule of energy in THREE separate transactions.

Ann-Louise Gittleson, PhD states that a "weak" Adrenal is a MAGNET for attracting Copper and is the biggest single CAUSE for its elevation in the body... Who knew?!?...

So, the PERFECT recipe for chronic disease is:

o   "Stress!" >> Mg deficiency

o   Adrenal Fatigue >> Low Mg-ATP (due to low Na and   Mg)

o   "Copper Toxicity" >> the perfect agent to oxidize and disrupt the cellular metabolism, and it does so silently and stealth fully -- never suspected by the client AND these three factors are NEVER discussed, nor measured by the practitioner... Hmmm...

Hope that sheds new light on the silent epidemic roiling thru MAG-land...

There are 12+ markers that correlate with "Copper Dysregulation" that have been developed by Paul Eck, PhD, Larry Wilson, MD, Michael McEvoy and other practitioners who have studied and worked with this medium to assess mineral optimal levels, and mineral metabolisum...

Type of Oxidizer	
Calcium	> 50
Sodium	< 12
Potassium	< 4
Copper	> 2.5
	< 1.5
Zinc	< 12
	> 20
Phosphorus	< 12
Ca/K ratio	> 10.1
Na/K ratio	< 2.1
Zn/Cu ratio	> 12:1
	< 6:1
Mercury (Hg) Level	> .02
Cu/Mo Ratio	> 625

Type of Oxidizer

2 or more Markers indicate a need for definitive blood testing. Tests that are recommended are as follows:

Magnesium RBC: best overall marker for metabolic health

Serum Copper: key mineral raised with weak Adrenals and low Mg-ATP

Plasma Zinc: essential antagonist for Copper, easily lost to "Stress!"

Serum Ceruloplasmin: Copper transport protein that also carries Iron

(Order tests: www.requestatest.com/mag-zinc-copper-panel-testing)

http://www.arltma.com/Mineral_Information/Copper.html

What the article says is when Na/K ratio is low (I.e. low Na and HIGH Potassium...) will respond to Copper, as Potassium will crash and Sodium will elevate slightly...

The key is discerning who has "Copper deficiency?!?"

o A "Fast" Oxidizer with a LOW Copper (Cu) likely has a deficiency...

o	A "Slow" oxidizer with a LOW Cu may have a metabolic Cu deficiency COUPLED with an excess of unbound (toxic) Copper...

And how do we attract Mo' Copper? Adrenal fatigue...

And how does Copper stay "unbound?" Lack of energy (Mg-ATP)

WHY is there a lack of energy? Adrenal Fatigue!

How did they get "Fatigued?!?" "Stressors!"

And what is LOST to "Stress!"?
Magnesium!

Hmmmmm...

Could it REALLY be that easy?!?

Whole food Vitamin-C Complex, has Copper enzymes at the core which are key to gaining access to bio-available Copper...

For the Copper "geek" set:

http://examine.com/supplements/Copper/

Please read slooooooowly to connect the dots with your condition(s) and likely under firing Copper enzymes...

Please read this one slooooooowly, as well:
http://www.holisticprimarycare.net/.../425-copper-deficiency

I'm also adding two of the more compelling references in this excellent article by Ronald Grabowski, RD, DC, a most talented and enlightened Chiropractor in the Houston, TX area
Hope it sheds important light on just how important this vilified mineral is…

Copper Deficiency May Underlie Osteoporosis, Anemia and Neurodegenerative Disorders :

http://www.holisticprimarycare.net/

Despite their obviously different appearances, osteoporosis, anemia, neuro-degenerative disorders, cardiovascular disease, and impaired cellular immunity may all be manifestations of chronic copper deficiency, an often-overlooked nutritional problem that is more common than many doctors realize.

The point of the article was to CLEARLY connect LACK OF BIOAVAILABLE COPPER to MOST of what ails ya!... It is a KEY Stealth Health issue…

Again, the focus is **NOT** on Copper, per se…

The focus IS on Ceruloplasmin (Cp) and the Liver's ability to make it sufficiently!

I was not suggesting SpectraCell as the way to assess this Cu/Cp dynamic. I do intend to chat with Dr. Grabowski this week to see how he measures Cp, and other relevant factors…

Please take 5 minutes to reflect on this excellent article on Copper co-authored by my Cupro-hero, Leslie M. Klevay, MD, PhD:

http://m.advances.nutrition.org/content/2/6/520.full.pdf

Now, here's the deal...

I'd like you to take 15 min to reflect on the following:

o   The 2nd sentence states: "Copper deficiency is the
        leading deficiency worldwide among nutritional diseases
        of agricultural animals."

Hmmmmmmmmm...

o   That sentence should send a chill down your
        spine... as great sources of Copper are eggs, pork
        products, lamb, goat, etc. Interesting that these were
        taken out of our diet 60 years ago... And yet we're told in
        article, after article, after article that the chance of Copper
        deficiency is RARE in humans... (*TILT!*)

o   In the paragraph on "Deficiencies," please read it
        slooooooowly as it explains HOW lack of
        bioavailable Copper is behind most, if not ALL, chronic
        diseases... ALL of those processes noted are the result
        of Cupro-enzymes NOT working   for LACK of
        bioavailable Copper...

o   "Adequate Copper intake permits normal utilization of
        dietary Iron in that intestinal iron absorption, iron release
        from stores (e.g. macrophages of liver and spleen), and
        iron incorporation into hemoglobin are COPPER-
        DEPENDENT [emphasis added!] process. Know
        anybody struggling with "Anemia?..."

Hmmmmmm...

o   "Inadequate Copper produces adverse effects on the
     metabolism of cholesterol and blood glucose, blood
     pressure control and heart function, mineralization of
     bones, and immunity." You mean high cholesterol, high
     blood pressure, heart disease, and osteoporosis ALL
     share the SAME mineral deficiency?....

HOW does Copper become deficient, or more accurately said:
"bio-UNavailable" in the Human animal?...

Unresolved "Stressors!"

As you well know, chronic "Stress!" depletes Maggie, and the
rise of "Stress!" Hormones ACTH>>Cortisol (made entirely from
Cholesterol mind you...) affect the production of Ceruloplasmin
(Cp) in the Liver which is the KEY protein essential for making
Copper bioavailable... High Cortisol = LOW Cp!

NOW, please ask your yourself the following questions:

o   When was the last time your Mineral Denialist assessed
     your Mag RBC?...or asked what the "Stress!" levels are in
     your life that might be depleting your Mg levels daily, not
     the least of which are the Rx meds that they have you
     taking, for conditions induced by Mg deficiency.

o   When was the last time your Mineral Denialist   assessed
     your Copper/Cp status?... or let you know the FACTS of
     the importance of Copper to run the human metabolism as
     noted in Klevay's article...

If the answer is NEVER, you might want to re-read this article AGAIN, and think about a NEW approach to addressing your metabolic dysfunction(s) that are ENTIRELY CAUSED by mineral deficiencies, and mineral dysregulation...

These "Labels" are NOT medical diseases... that is patently obvious from the research literature and its high time you start acting on that scientific reality...

There is not one person that is deemed "Copper Toxic" that isn't ALSO dealing with Copper deficiency... Beware the practitioners seeking to suck you dry of Copper... The focus needs to be on creating MORE Ceruloplasmin, to ACTIVATE that Copper -- NOT depleting elevations of Copper... in my humble opinion.

Please note the discussion of Copper<>Ascorbic Acid... It very clearly states the affect that this ubiquitous element (AA) has on Ceruloplasmin and Copper... this is found on pages 1057S-1058S for those whose Mg levels are sufficient enough to work their way through this excellent, but somewhat ponderous article...

It doesn't get more Black and White than this;

http://www.ncbi.nlm.nih.gov/pubmed/17236184

Note the TITLE says it ALL...

While Cuprum Metallicum is a wonderful intervention, I would advise a bit more testing to understand WHY your Copper may be bio-UNavailable...

What I'm sharing here, should be taught in TWO locations;

o Kindergarten, AND

o Medical Schools

And the more we do the former, the less we need the latter...

Just so you know... my read of the tea leaves seems to indicate that hemochromatosis is CAUSED by a Lack of Ceruloplasmin (Cp) and thus the body, in its infinite wisdom, knows to store the unbound Iron so that it doesn't do MORE damage in its unbound state...

The KEY to understanding your Copper dynamics is to KNOW your Ceruloplasmin (Cp) status... The tests that I routinely do for clients that are dealing with Copper-related issues, which is the BULK of my clientele, are the following;

o Mag RBC...
o Plasma Zinc...
o Serum Copper...
o Serum Ceruloplasmin...

http://requestatest.com/mag-zinc-copper-panel-testing

For those that are struggling with Iron/Anemia, I add the Serum Iron, Serum Transferrin, TBIC, % saturation and Serum Ferritin to see what's really cooking there... Again, as noted in the article above, the entire metabolism of Iron is COPPER DEPENDENT...

Request A Test MgZn-Copper panel whith these panels.

The Cu RBC is MOST helpful to know the status of your CuZnSOD which is the backbone of your anti-oxidant defense system. That RBC level of Copper is 60+% SOD... Why Minerals

Denialists DON'T know this, or know its importance is baffling beyond words...

Last licks, please know that elevated Cholesterol is a clinical sign of Copper deficiency, that was clearly established by Leslie M. Kelvay, MD, PhD in the early 1970's -- Yes, that is about the time $tain$ were introduced...
http://ajpendo.physiology.org/content/298/1/E138

You might print this out for your Cardiologist so that s/he can learn how the human body REALLY works...

Guess what?...

It's TRUE for EVERYONE'S Family Tree... Within mine, heart disease, rampant blood pressure, GB removals, kidney disease, cancer, manic-depression, etc... ALL connected to "Stress!"-induced Mg loss >> Copper dysregulation...

It's humbling to learn the mineral induced foundation of there dynamics...

Copper is tricky...

You really need to know whether you're a "Fast" or "Slow" Oxidizer... Fast's can take Copper supplements directly, Slows need to do so indirectly, with wholefood Vit-C... (If Slows take copper, it can push them into even slower state.)

Without knowing your Mag RBC, your Zinc or your Ceruloplasmin, as well as your Iron status, it's very difficult to comment. But since you asked...

Your protocol appears to be "attacking" the Copper, which is a common trend...

o   2:1 Calcium to Mag means you don't absorb any Mg...

o   Ascorbic Acid (Vit C) is intended to lower Copper but it will separate Copper from Cp, thus lowering the oxidise function of Cp, which is a PARAMOUNT function for Cp!..

o   Molybdenum is directly going to chelate Copper...

I see the dynamic differently.

What is being done to RESTORE/REBUILD the status of Ceruloplasmin production in your Liver?...

I see nothing in this protocol that is designed to do that...

Actually, this alternative focus makes more sense when you realize that SOD (SuperOxide Dismutase) is the BACKBONE of the AOD (Anti-Oxidant Defense) system...

What's the KEY to a STRONG and EFFECTIVE AOD?...

Copper bioavailability made possible by optimal levels of Cp! It's really quite easy when you STOP seeing Copper as a toxin and START realizing how important it is to run the human metabolism..

The fact that your Mineral Denialist has NEVER talked about, nor tested the critical componets and dynamics should alarm and enrage you...

Yes, it's THAT important!...

Please know that if you have Copper dysregulation issues, it's almost a certainty you've got Iron dysregulation issues as well. Furthermore, it's a lock your children do, as well... Apples never fall far from the tree...

I believe Copper and Iron dysregulations are involved in:

o   Salicylates...
o   Oxalates...
o   Nitrates...
o   Amines...
o   Sulfation...

Largely due to a lack of Anti-Oxidant enzymes (SOD and CAT) and lack of KEY Oxidase enzymes that neutralize the above ^^^^

Pretty amazing when you stop to think about HOW MANY people suffer for lack of bioavailability of this powerhouse mineral, Copper...

And chronic lack of Maggie undermines Copper's usefulness...

2 reasons:

1)   The body STOPS making Cp when we get too "Stressed!" (Elevated ACTH, and Cortisol) and

2)   Proper folding of the Cp protein (1,046 Amino Acids) requires Maggie.

Remember:

1)   Wiki is NOT a reliable source of scientific info...

2) There is a hot debate with the Copper community re Cu and Cp. There is a camp stating that there are 8 Cu ions -- I've no idea how that affects the   math of "estimating" usable Copper...

3) The production of Cp rests SOLELY in the Liver. The notion that "Adrenals affect Cp" stems from the fact that ACTH and/or Cortisol STOP the production of Cp. The Adrenals do NOT produce Cp. They DO produce "Stress!" hormones that can STOP Cp production...

4) It is worth noting that the synthesis of GSH requires Mg-ATP in 2 key places... Selenium is important, but don't forget, NOTHING happens without Maggie... Also, GSH in a Cu deficient body (that would be just about ALL of us...) does not work as well...

5) Metallothionein is important, but I'm just starting to set my sights there. There's no question it's a key protein, but I can't sort out its role with Copper -- YET! I don't know that it has enzymatic properties like Cp, though... Cp serves as a major anti-oxidant!

6) Weight of Mg = 24. The weight of Cu = 63.5. The weight of Hg = 200 Mercury is the Suma Wrestler of the body. I look forward to watching that video. Its reach and disruption is humbling...

7) My early research indicates that Hg behaves differently in the presence of CuZnSOD -- not an insignificant fact.

Here's how I would explain it...

o   The Mg in the HTMA is surrounded by a wide   spectrum of minerals. The real value of the HTMA is that it reveals the "Stress!" pattern of the individual, and how well they are mobilizing energy in the face of that "Stress!" -- These are profoundly important measures to have.

o   The Mg in the HTMA can be evaluated in terms of the Calcium level (to assess Blood Sugar and broad level of Stress), the Sodium level (to assess the Adrenal Ratio: Na/Mg), and micrometals and heavy metals in relation to the Mg...

o   The Mag RBC is an acid-test for "Stress!" and the potential for Inflammation, Oxidative Stress, etc.

Copper: Unusable Copper

Usable Copper depends upon healthy absorption of Copper in the Tummy (good stomach acid...) AND production of Ceruloplasmin (Cp) in the Liver, which feeds off:

o   Healthy "Stress!" Response (not excess ACTH due to Mg deficiency)

o   LACK OF THE Cp BLOCKERS:
        - LOW Retinol CAUSED by excess Storage-D supps!
        - excess Ascorbic Acid! (It's EVERYWHERE "Citric Acid!")
        - Excess HFCS...
        - Excess Glyphosate exposure
        -       Excess Zinc!- excess Calcium that BLOCKS absorption...
        -       Excess Iron that SHUTS DOWN Copper metabolism...Again, addressing Mg shortages is akin to arithmetic... Copper, however, is akin to Simultaneous Equations on Steroids...

Sorry!...

Folks, I'm really not trying to be evasive...

I think I've demonstrated beyond any measure of doubt where my intentions are...

The issue here is NOT just about Copper... It is VITAL to understand your Ceruloplasmin, your Zinc and your Iron levels, as well...

If REQUIRES proper, targeted testing to accurately assess what field of play of Copper/Iron/Zinc dynamics you're in. It is NOT necessarily about getting a "killer" form of Copper supplement.

Regrettably, it is NOT that straight-forward, and if a practitioner says it is, then smile, thank them for their time, turn around and slowly LEAVE their office. They simply do NOT get it, if their approach is to "ATTACK" the Copper... please re-read and repeat the comments ^^^^...

All we can do is continue to heal ourselves, allow our bodies and minds to become Billboards, and then more will follow...
For the most part, sheeple live in fear; and what they are MOST afraid of is

1)   The responsibility for taking care of themselves, and
2)   Having to change their lifestyle...

And not everyone is willing to expand their consciousness -- and that's OK... So, we bless them and move on!

Iodine: Factors To Consider

What I would advise is as follows:

o   Read the book by Lynne Farrow...The Iodine Crisis. It's
       outstanding!...

o   Heed David's advice on building the foundation, first --
       BEFORE taking the Iodine dive, but know that Lynne's the
       Iodine expert and I defer to her wisdom here. That said,
       my clients' who've responded to Iodine   the best have
       had optimal RBC Mg and RBC Selenium levels...

o   Assess your Mg RBC, Zinc, Copper and Ceruloplasmin
       status to assess the bioavailability of your Copper in your
       body. And if you've got Iron issues, please get them
       measured, as well...

o   If you've had dental work done in the recent past, it
       would be important to assess the extent to which
       Mercury may be a factor in disrupting your Copper and
       Iron metabolism which it LOVES to do...

That's enough to keep you off the streets for the next few weeks,
and as you have questions, don't hesitate to ask away!...

Iron: Factors To Consider

More to come in Musing From MAG!!! Vol III

IRON my spider sense tingles wildly when I hear client, after client, after client, after client is told that they are "Iron Anemic!" 90% of the time, ALL the doctor did was look at Ferritin, which is HIGHLY sensitive to Copper status...

In the SAME way that folks are savvy about how to assess Thyroid function BEYOND just TSH, I would advise the following to truly understand "Iron status":

- **Serum Iron**
- **Serum Transferrin**
- **TIBC**
- **% Sat**
- **Serum Copper**
- **Serum Ceruloplasmin (it is ESSENTIAL for proper Iron metabolism...)**
- **Plasma Zinc (Iron and Zinc have a wicked relationship**
- **Mag RBC**

And if the individual is taking Calcium supplements or Calcium on Steroids (Vitamin-D), well then ALL bets are off, as Calcium BLOCKS Iron absorption -- which too few practitioners take into account when making the "AD" (Anemia Declaration!)
Food for thought...

ALL MAG-pies... Please read the following excerpt on Copper to BETTER understand the issues of Iron Metabolism:

http://lpi.oregonstate.edu/mic/minerals/copper

Please pay particular attention to the Section on Iron Metabolism in that overview ^^^^, and note the 2nd sentence of that piece: "Anemia is a clinical sign of Copper deficiency..."

Please be sure to re-read that sentence AGAIN...

That is NOT a typo coming from the great Linus Pauling Institute. I have seen that EXACT same phrase in a dozen snooty scientific articles. Yes, it is WELL KNOWN on the Research side of Medical Education- - from anemia is a COPPER issue...

There is NO aspect of Iron Metabolism that is not RULED by the bioavailability of Copper... And what GUARANTEES that? The optimal production of Ceruloplasmin (Cp)!

And what BLOCKS Cp production FLAWLESSLY? Paying attention to conventional idiocy re the need for Iron supplements that is routinely pushed by the Mineral Denialist agents of BIG Pharma...

Let go of your phobia re Iron deficiency... shift your focus to ensuring bioavailable Copper and you'll come into the light...

A FAAAAR more likely CAUSE of poor Iron absorption is excess Calcium and excess Calcium-on-Steroids, aka Hormone-D, and the belief that Copper is TOXIN!!!.

Please note, Calcium BLOCKS Iron absorption in the gut...

An easily overlooked mechanism is the proverbial "Green Smoothie" stuffed with Spinach and loads of Phytates!...

69

In fact, the Multi-Copper Oxidase (MCO) Hephaestin, which requires 4 Copper ions to work, is ESSENTIAL for Iron absorption in the gut...

Where, oh where, would we find four (4) Copper ions regularly?!? In each molecule of wholefood Vit-C!

Liver is HIGH in Vit-A, needed for Cp production, and has a balance of Cu<>Zn<>Fe... It is NOT just Iron.

Blood builder is a very cool product that, again, offers a spectrum of nutrients, especially Manganese (Mn) that has a special relationship with Copper!

Many MAG-pies have had excellent results focusing on the combo of wholefood Vit-C + Blackstrap Molasses... Again, Molasses has a spectrum of minerals, NOT just Iron...

Given all that effort, it would be advisable to assess how well you're making Cp, as Mo' Iron and LOW Cp is a wicked combo!!!

Apparently, the metabolic requirement that Iron has for Copper is getting lost...

Yes, the Iron is actually OK, but the THREE Cu-dependent Iron proteins are Low: Ferritin, TIBC and %Sat...

Hmmmm...

Now why would that be?...

Maybe because there's a serious shortage of USABLE Copper?...

And that's EXACTLY what's here:

o   Mag is at the BOTTOM of the Range...

o   Zinc is Below optimum...

o   Usable Copper (3X Cp) is Below optimum...

o   Zn:Usable Copper is below what it should be 1.2...

o   Potassium RBC is ALSO at the bottom...

Bottom line: there's work to be done to restore Mg, Zn and Cp status...

The WORST thing you could do would be to take supplemental Iron as doctors suggest... And why is that?!?

It will shut down your Copper metabolism and drive your Anemia even deeper!

The ENTIRE Iron Metabolism is DEPENDENT on bioavailable Copper. Scientists have KNOWN this since ~1860, on the research side of medicine... Not so, on the Clinical side of medicine...

Ceruloplasmin (Cp) is a critical protein that brings life to BOTH Copper and Iron. (In Iron research circles, this very protein is called Ferroxidase -- but it's the EXACT same protein...)

What's the most PERFECT way to bring the Liver's production of Cp to its knees?...

Take ridiculous doses of unopposed Hormone-D!... (Know anybody "D"oing that?!?...) And/or take supplemental Iron in response to a misleading "LOW" ferritin blood test.

I've identified 20+ steps that are needed to RESTORE Cp function in a body that has been following "D"aily "D"ietary "D"ictums...

Steps to Increase Ceruloplasmin (Cp):

o STOP Hormone-D ONLY Supplements (KILLS Liver Retinol needed for Cp)
o STOP Calcium Supplements! (Ca BLOCKS Mg & Iron absorption...)
o STOP Iron Supplements! (Fe SHUTS DOWN Cu metabolism...)
o STOP Ascorbic Acid (It disrupts the Copper<>Cp bond)
o STOP HFCS & Synthetic Sugars (HFCS Lowers Liver Copper)
o STOP LOW Fat Diet (Fat is needed for proper Copper absorption)
o STOP Using Industrialized, "Heart Healthy" Oils!
o STOP Using products w/ Fluoride (toothpaste, bottled Water, etc.)
o STOP Taking "Mulit's" & "Pre-natals" (They have 1st four items ^^^^)

o START CLO (1 tsp Rosita's or 1 TBSP Nordic Naturals) for Retinol (Vit-A)
o START Mg supps to lower ACTH & Cortisol (Dose: 5mgs/lb body weight)
o START Wholefood Vit-C (500-800 mgs/day) - source of Copper
o START B8 (Biotin) -- Key for Cu/Fe regulation in Liver
o START B2 (Riboflavin) -- Key for Cu/Fe regulation in Liver
o START Boron -- 1-3 mgs/day (aids in Synthesis of Cp)
o START Taurine to support Copper metabolism in the Liver
o START Ancestral Diet (HIGH Fat & Protein/LOW Carb)
o START Iodine (PREQUISITE: Mg & Se RBC need to be optimal)

Please find a great chapter in my other Ebook "Let's Get Sick!"

Independent Source, MAG wall member: The Copper - Ceruloplasmin Connection and its influence on Iron metabolism Copper - (Cu) is an essential trace element for humans and animals. This trace element plays an important role as essential Co-factor in oxidation-reduction reactions and in scavenging free radicals. Its enzymes regulate various physiologic pathways like energy production, connective tissue maturation, and neurotransmission and iron metabolism.

Copper imbalance has been linked to impaired immune function, bone demineralization, and increased risk of cardiovascular and neuro-degenerative diseases. Further copper deficiency can also lead to secondary Ceruloplasmin deficiency and hepatic iron overload and/or cirrhosis.

Copper deficiency includes symptoms like central nervous system demyelination, polyneuropathy, myelopathy, and inflammation of the optic nerve. Dysfunctional copper metabolism is suggested as a risk factor for AD, it could also be symptomatic of the disease and it may play a role in Parkinson Disease too. Copper deficiency of bound Cu can further result in heart abnormalities because outside the body, free (unbound/ not bound to Ceruloplasmin) Copper is known to be a pro-oxidant. Iron - (Fe) is an essential trace element too and Fe-deficiency (anemia) is a clinical sign of Cu-imbalance/deficiency. It's indicating that more bio-available Copper (Cu bound to Ceruloplasmin) is required for Iron transport to the bone marrow for red blood cell formation. For adequate Iron metabolism four copper-containing enzymes (Multi-Copper-Oxidase) are required and the MCO family comprises the circulating Ceruloplasmin.

Ceruloplasmin – (Cp) is a ferroxidase enzyme (produced in the liver, which depends on Magnesium, real Vitamin C and animal based Vitamin A) that has the capacity to oxidize ferrous iron (Fe^{2+}) to ferric iron (Fe^{3+}), which can be loaded onto the iron-transport protein, transferrin. A lack in Ceruloplasmin displays iron overload in selected tissues, including liver, brain, and retina. The cuproenzymes, superoxide dismutase and Ceruloplasmin, are known to have antioxidant properties.

High supplemental Zinc intakes of 50mg/day or more for extended periods of time may result in copper deficiency because such intakes increase the synthesis of an intestinal cell protein called metallothionein, which binds certain metals and prevents their absorption by trapping them in intestinal cells causing a decrease in copper absorption.

LOW Magnesium and LOW wholefood Vitamin C and Retinol (animal based Vit-A) => LOW Ceruloplasmin (Cp) production => LOW amounts of bound/bio-available Copper => HIGH amounts of unbound/bio-unavailable Copper and Iron => toxic Copper and Iron storage in the liver or brain tissue=> HIGH pro-oxidant status of the body.

LOW Magnesium caused by HIGH Calcium (e.g. dramatically increased with synthetic Hormone D intake ("Calcium on steroids"!) => BLOCKS Iron absorption in the gut even further! Multi-Copper Oxidase (MCO) requires 4 Copper ions to work which are essential for Iron absorption. This process HAS TO HAVE enough whole food Vit- C, where it will get ALL of its SO MUCH needed Ions.

The Minerals/Trace elements: Magnesium -Calcium, Copper – Zinc –Iron and the Vitamins: Wholefood Vit-C, animal based A and all the Bs, best from MTHR nature.

http://lpi.oregonstate.edu/

I'm still working my way thru this "maze," but here's a rundown of some basics;

o   The Iron uptake enzyme in the gut is activated by Whole food Vit-C Complex (which itself is activated by Maggie...)

o   Ferroxidase, the Iron transport enzyme is activated by Mg-ATP...

o   Ferritin, the Iron storage protein is Mg-dependent... The higher the Mag RBC, the higher the Ferritin...

o   The enzymes to put Oxygen ONTO Hemoglobin are Mg dependent, as are the enzymes to take O2 off and put it in tissue are, as well...

o   The shape of the Red Blood Cell (bi-concave) is totally dependent on the amount of Mg-ATP to ensure proper shape, and thus optimal Oxygen carrying capacity...

o   Globulin, the base protein, can NOT be made without Mg...

So, tell me again why the "spotlight" is on Iron when it comes to "Anemia?!?" It's worth noting that FeSO4, the standard issue Iron supplement to "correct" Anemia is, in fact, toxic to the Liver, and consumes copious amounts of Mg to run Detox Pathway to clear it.

From what I've learned from clients, the ONE and ONLY aspect of metabolism that INCREASES when taking this Iron supplement is CONSTIPATION! - - A classic sign of Mg deficiency...

Getting the picture yet?!?...

Hmmm...

The conditioning of your mind is DEEP...

Iron and Copper are SIAMESE TWINS connected to Ceruloplasmin.

Isn't it interesting that you've been trained -- like Circus Bears -- to obsess over your Iron levels, but NEVER told that Copper is THE MINERAL that makes it work properly in the human body...

Again, this is ALL courtesy of the Affagato, Allopathetic Medical machine that delights in your REPEAT business, NOT your health independence...

And if you are using Ferritin as your sole measure of Iron status, that's akin to using TSH to assess your Thyroid...

Embrace the totality and breadth of what is involved in attaining optimal Iron and Copper balance...

The "Iron-y" with ALL the above ^^^^
is that insufficient quantities of Cp (Ceruloplasmin) is at the CORE...

That protein, which is ALSO called Ferroxidase I, plays a pivotal role keeping Iron from rusting you out! THAT'S why, in my humble opinion, the body is storing the Iron because it knows it lacks the Cp/Ferroxidasse to BIND IT!

And given the CENTRAL role of MAKING Heme with properly bound Cu, and that Hepcidin is Cu-dependent, I'm NOT buying the MSM BS that these are "genetic disorders..."

The process to turn genes "On" and "Off" requires methylation. And as far as I can tell, Methyltransferase enzymes, that enable the "On/Off" Switch aware ALSO Copper dependent... This has the APPEREANCE of a "gene defect," but it is TOTAL Allopathetic witchcraft, in my humble opinion.

I would STRONGLY recommend you get the Mag-Zn-Cu-Cp and Iron blood panel and get SMART on Cp and teach your Idiopath how the body REALLY works, especially the Zn<>Cu<>Fe mineral triangle...

Remember, you'll need measurements of BOTH Copper and Ceruloplasmin...

And you Iron, Ferritin, tranferrin, saturation and TIBC are essential to assess the bioavailability of Iron, and it's impact upon Copper...

Regrettably, there is NOTHING straight forward about Copper/Iron regulation...

Iron: It's Relation To Copper

Please read the following excerpt on Copper to BETTER understand the issues of Iron Metabolism:

http://lpi.oregonstate.edu/mic/minerals/copper

Please pay particular attention to the Section on Iron Metabolism in that overview ^^^^, and note the 2nd sentence of that piece: "Anemia is a clinical sign of Copper deficiency..."

Please re-read that sentence AGAIN...

That is NOT a typo coming from the great Linus Pauling Institute. I have seen that EXACT same phrase in a dozen snooty scientific articles. Yes, it is WELL KNOWN on the Research side of Medical Education...

There is NO aspect of Iron Metabolism that is not RULED by the bioavailability of Copper... And what GUARANTEES that? The optimal production of Ceruloplasmin (Cp)!

And what BLOCKS Cp production FLAWLESSLY? Paying attention to conventional idiocracy re the need for Iron supplements and Hormone-D, that is routinely pushed by the Mineral Denialist agents of BIG Pharma...

Let go of your phobia re Iron deficiency... shift your focus to ensuring bioavailable Copper and you'll come into the light...

LOW Ceruloplasmin (Cp) will force Iron storage. In the face of a HIGH Iron source, I.e. water, that is the body's ONLY option...

I would also wonder how sufficient your Copper status is given that the Liver MUST HAVE Copper to make Cp!

Iron and Copper here is my gift to ALL:

http://ac.els-cdn.com/S1.../1-s2.0-S1550413113000521-main.pdf

http://m.clinchem.org/content/43/8/1457.long

Mary Fields, Phd, is highly recognized researcher in Copper and Iron circles...

Please know that wholefood Vit-C has Copper ions which is the TRUE reason why Iron metabolism is so dependent on Vit-C, but NOT Ascorbic Acid, the anti-oxidant shell...

Robert Thompson - Remember, the human cannot use copper in its metabolism without a piece of the C molecule called Tyrosinase. There are many forms of tyrosinase enzymes in the human. But, the C molecule one is special and unique.

Obviously, ascorbic acid (not C) does not contain this all important enzyme. This simple fact and the last two posts by Morley, impressive articles on copper and metabolism in the human, explains much of the why and how the actual vitamin C molecule deficiency in the human is such an incredibly significant root cause of so many diseases and illnesses in the human.
It is really quite simple. When one ponders this, even for only a short time, it becomes overwhelming in significance.

The C molecule enables your body to utilize copper. If your body is C molecule deficient, e.g. from taking ascorbic acid over time, thereby depleting the whole C molecules from your body, normal copper utilization cannot take place and it can accumulate or not be utilized and be lost.

Diet and supplementation are certainly important issues, and I pay close attention to the actual copper levels on HTMA and make supplement and diet changes as are appropriate.
But in both cases, copper excess and deficiency, the C molecule is the key that unlocks the door to copper reassuming its vital role in our bodies connective tissue (this means all connective tissue, i.e. bones, cartilage, ligaments, fascia, arterial walls, and all healing), bruising and bleeding tendencies, blood clotting ability, cholesterol metabolism (the building block of all hormones and 25% of our brain), thyroid hormone production, insulin production and activity, haemoglobin synthesis, and the list could go on and on.

There is so much illness related to this issue that the entire health statistics of the world could be changed by simply recognizing this deception and making the appropriate correction. (Chapter 7, The Calcium Lie 2 speaks to these issues).

Minerals: How Does The Liver Process Minerals

It's a complicated answer... The Liver engages in hundreds/thousands of enzyme reactions. Personally, I'm no fan of Livestrong as a website, but this gives a decent overview:

http://www.livestrong.com/.../398419-the-vitamins.../...

As expected, this article grossly downplays Maggie's role in BOTH Phase II and Phase I Detox, as well as activation of the many vitamins noted, as well as Glucose metabolism, as well as the creation and energizing (via Mg-ATP in 2 places) of the Glutathione pathway...

Clearly, there are numerous minerals and vitamins involved. Lay and scientific literature lead you to believe that Mg is merely one of the nutrients... Not much happens in the Liver without energy -- NO Mg >> NO Energy >> NO Enzyme Action >> Dysfunctional Liver>>Mo' needed for detox!...

And please know that "Fatty Liver Disease" is purely CAUSED by mineral deficiency, especially Magnesium and Copper...

Molasses: Minerals Source - Factors To Consider

I'm not sure re the mineral content of this brand vs others out there. They DO differ significantly in their contents so it behooves you to compare. Note that Blackstrap Molasses contains Iron, and regular Molasses does NOT.

Here's an overview of the different grades (colors) of Molasses:

http://johndlee.hubpages.com/.../Light--Dark-or...

https://www.organicfacts.net/health-benefits/other/health-benefits-of-molasses.html

Potassium and Magnesium: Factors To Consider

Not what you want to hear, but Magnesium recovery is the recognized precursor...

http://www.ncbi.nlm.nih.gov/pubmed/3732091

What is key is to know the mineral status across the board, as represented in an HTMA which then allows you to support the Adrenals, as well, which usually involves Sodium and Potassium...

There is too much sugar in Bananas... I would focus on Potatoes or Sweet Potatoes, celery, Coconut Water, Apple Cider Vinegar, etc. for the Potassium punch...

MOST fruit in America has been hybridized to death, and has faaaaar more Sugar and faaaaaar less minerals than the same fruits our Ancestors ate, decades ago...

I know, I know, another shocking revelation...

You might want to check your urine pH 1st thing in the morning...

I wonder if your pH is low enough that it's creating a block in your uptake... just a hunch... You can get strips from your local Health Food Store or some pharmacies carry them, as well...

Cortisol becomes LOW because your Potassium is sub-basement... NOT a sustainable pattern. This is caused by chronic "Stress!" or wanton use of Hormone-D (a MAJOR metabolic "Stressor!")... And it is VERY difficult to assess TRUE Copper status without doing a targeted blood test to assess Mag RBC, Zn, Cu and Ceruloplasmin (Cp) the protein that makes Copper bioavailable, and its ability to produce Ferroxidase to make Iron usable as well...

These issues also show in an HTMA which warrants further attention. Too bad your doctor doesn't understand mineral metabolism -- the FOUNDATION of human metabolism...

So what does it mean if potassium shows up high on a HTMA? It's all relative...

o   If you're a Fast Oxidizer and Na is elevated, all's likely normal...

o   If you're a Slow oxidizer, it could signal some "Stressor!" Is causing a Loss of Potassium...

o   It really can only be interpreted in the context of all the other minerals, especially the Electrolytes, and the transition metals like Copper, and from that can affect K status...

There are NO absolutes in HTMA interpretation... Context is KING!

It is easily identified with an HTMA (hair tissue mineral analysis). It is the ratio of Calcium/Phosphorus as expressed in the hair that dictates which way you're oxidizing the Electrolytes...

o   Slows hold onto the "Slow" minerals – Calcium and Magnesium...

o   Fasts hold onto the "Fast" minerals -- Sodium and Potassium It also has to do with our metabolic relationship with Copper, but FB doesn't have enough bandwidth to get into THAT discussion...

VITAMINS

Choosing your Supplements

Did we ever think we'd have to be THIS CAUTIOUS selecting supplements in our entire life...

And as I've said before, and WILL say again, and again, and again...

Where is the FDA in all this madness?!?...

Don't worry, I've NOT lost it... I'm presenting that as PURELY a rhetorical question...

Whole Food Source is where it's at!!!!

Cod Liver Oil - CLO

In order to get the desired benefit from Cod Liver Oil, it should contain 10 parts Vit-A (retinol) and 1 part Vit-D...

When I am choosing Cod Liver Oil, I am mindful of what my great-grandmother got...

Here's the breakdown of some leading brands and what I look for are products that deliver a MUCH HIGHER ratio of Vit-A to Hormone-D:

Vit-A to Hormone-D Ratio

o   Great-grandmother's CLO 5,000:400 10:1, Brand of CLO
o   Carlson (bottle) 850:400 ~2:1
o   Carlson (tabs) 150:80 ~2:1
o   Nordic Naturals (bot) 2,950:20 147:1
o   Nordic Naturals (tab) 1,770:12 147:1
o   Standard Process 2,000:90 ~ 22:1
O   Rosita's Extra Virgin 2,000:90 ~ 22:1

Based on this analysis, I personally take SP and recommend Rosita's and Nordic Naturals-Artic, only because so many folks have difficulty finding/getting SP products...

The body needs a healthy dose of Vitamin-A (retinol), especially to keep the Hormone-D in check -- despite all the silly articles that you've read about how "D"eficient we are!...

Cod Liver Oil - Why it's the key

Is it just me, or are others exhausted beyond belief with the ENDLESS "D"eception and "D"istortion that permeates this "FISHY" industry!!!

I'm tempted to "D"rink with NO restraint!!!!!

Oy vey…

;-(

http://www.dailymail.co.uk/news/article-55564/Why-cod-liver-oil-really-good-you.html

Folks, that is NOT Rocket Science…

o   CLO has a significant infusion of Retinol, animal-based Vit-A that is ESSENTIAL in the production of Ceruloplasmin (Cp)…

o   Optimal levels of Cp = Optimal levels of bioavailable Copper = Optimal levels of Anti-Oxidant Enzymes/Cuproenzymes/NORMAL metabolic function…

o   Bioavailable Copper -- properly bound to its INTENDED protein, Cp -- is a wonder inside the body, inside the cell, and inside the Mitochondria…

o   Bioavailable Copper STOPS Oxidative Stress in its tracks...

o   Oxidative Stress, we know it as "RUST," is VERY TOXIC to the cells' vitality and vibrancy…

When was the last time your Mineral Denialist MEASURED your Anti-Oxidant Defense status?!?…

Or do they just wring their hands and teach you to just "deal with" your growing litany of symptoms INDUCED by Oxidative Stress?!?…

HOW in the world do they stand it?!?…

WHY in the world do we tolerate this kind of INCOMPETENCE?!

Ratio matters 10:1 – Retinol:Vit-D

Musings of Mg Man on a fine am...

Fat Soluble Vitamins

There is a HEAVY price to the moronic, "D"emonic, nutritionally FLAWED protocol of the "LOW FAT" diet... Our tissues are severely parched for Fat Soluble Vitamins, especially A and E...

And HOW do we do that?!?...

OBSESS about D and K, in isolation of their lipid-loving partners...

There are FOUR Fat Soluble Vitamins: A, D, E, and K... I find it entertaining that we are pummelled to "D"eath to take D and K -- but SILENCE on A and E...

I've learned to hold a mirror up to conventional "D"irectives and DO THE OPPOSITE!...

Hope you're O"K" with that...

There is NO benefit in "micro-dosing" a BAD product... Please place it in your "round file!"

Factoids of Depletion:

The generational depletion of minerals has been building for the last 100 years -- thanks to:

o   Commercial farming (fertilizers, pesticides and mono-
         cropping to extreme...)

o   Food processing that has introduced thousands of food
         chemical never before seen in food...

o   Water treatment that introduces Aluminium and
         Fluoride, among many other toxins...

o   Dental practices that obsess about "teeth" and IGNORE
         the obvious toxic effect of Fluoride and Mercury...

o   The global domination of GMO seed and Glyphosate --
         designed for end game annihilation...

o   An Affagato, Allopathetic Medical machine that values
         suppression of symptoms via toxic, mineral-depleting
         synthetic drugs...

We are the 4th-5th generation of depletion... It is VERY real. It is
correctable, but it requires MASSIVE change on a personal and
global level. Most are unaware or unwilling to pay that price...

All we can do is address the issues within our personal sphere of
influence. It is a day-by-day battle...

Alas... Too many people have been "programmed" to believe this Nursery Rhyme:

"Jack Sprat could eat no fat, His wife could eat no lean; and so betwixt them both, They lick'd the platter clean."

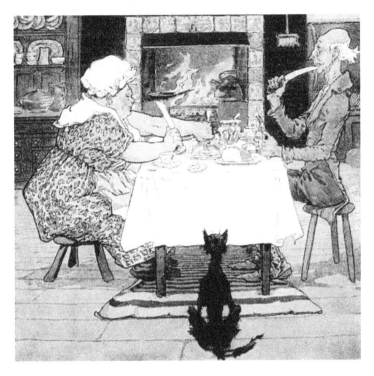

When it comes to Lipids, Chris Masterjohn, PhD is a "rock star!"

He is smart, funny, penetrating and impeccably trained -- a killer combo that will unnerve the conventional establishment types.

Haven't read this one in a while, but please know that the fat soluble vitamins: A, D, E, and K ALL have a relationship with the Electrolytes (Ca, Mg, Na, and K) and they are the medium that is key to the movement of those minerals...

Best source of these 4 vitamins?... Unprocessed milk from your favorite Dairy Farmer down the street...

(Said another way, the LAST place you'll find them is in the "white liquid" that you think is "milk" at the store...) And short of that, grass-fed butter from cows allowed to graze in the sun!

The 3 Metal Amigos In Harmony Zn<>Cu<>Fe

There's nothing like adding bioavailable Copper -- properly balanced with Zinc and Iron -- to enhance the body's stores of this vital nutrient…

I once asked one of the world's authorities on Copper, Leslie M. Klevay, MD, PhD, what the BEST source of Copper/Zinc/Iron was? His response:

Grass-fed Beef Liver! (There was NO hesitation in his response...)

He did NOT say chicken livers, duck or goose...

I checked the nutrient databases for these four forms and found that the BALANCE of the Zinc/Copper/Iron was decidedly different in BEEF than the fowl...

Maybe THAT'S why our Ancestors had Beef Liver 3-4X each month...

Wholefood C: Ascorbic Acid debate

I've just ordered this book:

https://www.amazon.com/.../ref=od_aui_detailpages00...

Which I read about here:

http://www.alternativemedicine.com/.../can-you-%E2%80%9Cc...

I believe "Ascorbate" is STILL Ascorbic Acid WITHOUT the critical factors...

The paragraph towards the end re Sherry Lewin, PhD seems to imply that there is MUCH missing from the "Ascorbic Acid" -- most notably the Copper ions which are KEY to the functions that are described in that section of this article...

One question folks...

Where does the Copper ion come from that is ESSENTIAL to make Ascorbate Oxidase enzyme work?...

That is WHY we need this Vitamin and that is WHY the Wholefood molecule is SOOOOO important...

Please, get beyond the banal debate of Ascorbic Acid and ask yourself, "so HOW does the enzyme associated with this VITAL anti-oxidant Vital amine REALLY work?!?..."

And if you think it's coming from inside your body, think again...

Vitamin C is NOT Ascorbic Acid because real "C" has six parts to it, one being Copper ions, know that Ascorbic Acid does increases the separation of Copper from its protein "Ceruloplasmin" and to much unbound Copper is very taxing to Mg, Zn and B6 = toxic to our bodies, which is "simple" Bio-chemistry so to speak.

Tyrosinase is the precursor to Melanin... This is yet another Cu-dependent process, as are MOST of the biosynthetic pathways of Neurotransmitters...

Please don't be *fooled* by the literature that hypes several of these enzymes being "Iron dependent..." If Copper ain't happy, there's NO WAY for Iron to be happy. They are joined at the hip of Ceruloplasmin (Cp)!

Again, Tyrosinase is found at the center of the wholefood Vit-C Complex...

Given all that, what then is your question?...

There are about a thousand regulatory functions directed by Mg and Mg-ATP...

o   There is a key role that Mg-ATP plays in activating the Na/K ATPase pumps in EVERY cell of the body to keep Na outside and Potassium inside the cell...

o   It plays a pivotal role to PREVENT the conversion of Angiotensin I >> Angiotensin II, which is what ACE Inhibitors are designed to do synthetically, but the Rx Meds CAUSE Mg LOSS (No, that is NOT a typo)...

o   It also LOWERS Stress Hormones which then enable the increased production of Ceruloplasmin (Cp) in the Liver, which enables MORE bioavailable Copper and thus INCREASED SOD enzyme to LOWER Oxidative Stress which is at the heart of Hypertension... That's   just 3 of the MANY roles for Maggie...

Mg LOWERS "Stress!" which lowers BP... Mg has a keen regulatory role to keep Na and K in optimal balance...

Most folks with High BP have excess Na and too little K... If hospitals gave Mg IVs they would have FAR MORE empty beds...

Mg regulates... That is its primary metabolic role in the body, much to the chagrin and confusion of conventional practitioners the world over...

Most folks with POTS have dysregulated Copper. Copper plays a key role to help elevate Na in the body... If you're relying on Allopathetic types to sort out your minerals, I'd think again on that approach...

Are you aware of ANY studies that have assessed the impact on Ceruloplasmin (Cp) by IVs of:

o   Ascorbic Acid?!?
o   Sodium or other Ascorbates?!?
o   Liposomal Ascorbic Acids?!?

Given that Ascorbic Acid destroys BOTH Ceruloplasmin bioavailability and Tyrosinase functionality, what is the longer-term impact of this acute intervention?...

My intent was most sincere... I have NO studies up my sleeve...

This is NOT an "academic" argument -- at all. I wonder MIGHTILY where practitioners think all the Copper is coming from to fire up the infusion of the catalyst for Ascorbate Oxidase, which is ENTIRELY Copper dependent AND I worry MIGHTILY about the back-end impact this infusion has on Ceruloplasmin (Cp)?!?...

In my humble opinion, it is an ENTIRELY appropriate set of questions to consider for a profession whose ignorance of and arrogance re the central role of minerals in human metabolism invites anger and NOT the humility that seems justly warranted...

Please know, Copper is akin to a Violin... It's "status" is PROFOUNDLY affected when the Bow (Ceruloplasmin) is made smaller, or in actuality, disappears!

http://www.jbc.org/content/238/5/1675.full.pdf

The RDA for:

o   Ascorbic Acid = 1,000mgs
o   Wholefood C = 60mgs

It is "social construction of reality" that we believe we need MASSIVE doses of an INFERIOR form of this vital agent to work... If people really understood HOW IMPORTANT bioavailable Copper is to optimal health and immune function, they would NEVER go near Ascorbic Acid again...

I suppose you could combine lecithin with something like Pure Radiance "Alive!" to make a Liposomal wholefood C. I've no idea how that would work...

I listened to ~45 min of Humphries lecture on "C" -- she is NEITHER "brilliant," NOR accurate! And she is hardly comfortable with public speaking...

Regrettably, she is more like a Circus/Carnival Barker with 3 Walnut Shells and a pea moving haphazardly from:

o   Wholefood Vit-C (she ACTUALLY uses the term...)

o	Sodium Ascorbate, and

o	Ascorbic Acid... But she leaves the listener with the distinct impression they are ALL the same. That is patently FALSE and completely misleading... This was MOST disheartening lecture!

And to add insult to injury, she then proceeds to connect "Vit-C" to many Key Enzymes that are FOR A FACT, COPPER DEPENDENT... like Lysyl Oxidase or Ceruloplasmin...

She NEVER reveals the mineral foundation for any of these critical enzymes and she completely fails to explain the structure of "Vit-C" to reveal that it is, FOR A FACT, the source of these vital Copper ions needed in those enzymes...

Why is this SOOOOO difficult for physicians to grasp these mineral concepts?!?...

So we are left hanging by this "C"onfusing, "C"onvoluted and "C"on founding dis"C"ourse...

Were I grading it, she would earn a "C-"

And in that same vein, what's wrong with supplement companies coming clean with folks and telling them the TRUTH for a change about this vital supplement...

Why is THAT soooooo hard?...

It's ever so much more profitable to keep the Masses in the dark like Mushrooms and have quick witted spokesmen dispel their nostrums of "D"eceit and "D"eception...

Why change a business model that has worked for the last century?...

Are we talking about Ascorbic Acid or wholefood Vit-C?...

The latter has the Tyrosinase enzyme at its CORE and each Tyrosinase enzyme has FOUR (4) atoms of Copper...

Are these critters REALLY helping to create THAT?!?...

The issue is NOT Ascorbic Acid...

It's the body's ability to execute and benefit from Ascorbate Oxidase function.

Enzymatic Assay of ASCORBATE OXIDASE (EC 1.10.3.3) PRINCIPLE: 2 L-Ascorbic Acid + O2>> (Ascorbate Oxidase)>>> 2L- Dehydroascorbic Acid + 2 H2O

That enzymatic reaction will NOT happen without bioavailable Copper...

http://www.jbc.org/content/248/19/6596.full.pdf

That article ^^^ suggests that it doesn't matter whether it's Cuprous (Cu+) or Cupric (Cu2+), but I'm increasingly of the opinion that it's the FORMER that works MAG-ic in our bodies. Or as Charles Barker likes to say: "Proper" Copper has a valence of 1+!"

I would advise moving away from this exploration of Ascorbic Acid and focus on how this vitamin, and many other vitamins and enzymes are LOST without "Proper" Copper...

That we're just figuring this out is a bit disheartening, but we ARE figuring it out and the world of convention had best step aside as we now know the game and will not tolerate the "D"eception any more...

As I'm coming to learn it, Copper that is complexed with KEY enzymes like: Tyrosinase, Ceruloplasmin, Cytochrome c Oxidase, and ALL Oxidase enzymes for that matter, are using "Proper" Copper...

Where we get into BIG issues of dysregulation and dysfunction is that we are "D"rowning in Copper that has been attached to anions with a 2+ valence (like $CuSO_4$ that is sprayed on produce, and water treatment plants as an anti-fungal...), which means that Copper is, in fact, Cupric... And that rhymes with "Toxic!" -- which it is, especially when there's NOT enough of the enzymes noted above^^^^ to make Copper behave...

OMg! Please WAKE UP!

We are living POST-1984!

Yes, there is a "They!" and they "D"elight in "D"issension and "D"ebate! In fact, they want us to "D"ie for it!... (Get it?!?) I LOVE that you're researching and questioning... It's what MAG is ALL about.

But DO REAL RESEARCH! Get beyond the facade of polite internet articles that are dishing out re-hashed Pablum... Dig in and study the following:

o   How Iron fortification is THE agent of metabolic chaos...

o   How the US, UK, and Canada are the ONLY 3 nations in the Western world that FORTIFY IRON... Hmmmm...

(You might study the incidence of chronic disease in the US, UK, and Canada, vs the rest of the Western world...)

o   Yes, that Ascorbic Acid does increase the absorption of Iron, but at WHAT COST?!?...

o   That Ascorbic Acid increases the action of Aconitase...

o   That Aconitase is now recognized as a MAJOR source of Fe^{2+} and H_2O_2 -- that is NOT something to get excited about!

o   That increased Ferritin Iron is tied to Oxidative Stress!

o   That Oxidative Stress is THE battleground in aging and chronic disease.

o   That ALL 3 Anti-Oxidant Enzymes, SOD, CAT, GSH have KEY and KEEN relationships with Copper.

o   That Tyrosinase enzyme is WAAAAAAAAY more important than what Wikipedia or the Pablum-focused research is "training" you to believe... (When you seen "Tyrosinase," think Tyrosine...

More Hmmmmmmmm...)
Royal Lee, DDS, founder of Standard Process, was a genius. And that's a fact!

That said, he developed his amazing array of food concentrates 75 years BEFORE the toxic assault of Monsanto, BIG Pharma, FDA, etc. The hit to our mineral status has been devastating, esp. to Mg and Copper (found INSIDE the Tyrosinase found INSIDE the wholefood Vit-C Complex.)

Best approach, take both... 95% of the body's stores of Vit-C are found in our Adrenals... Feed them! They are undernourished, and that, too, is a fact!

Unfortunately, folks, I would strongly encourage you to tune up your BS Filters and start bucking up to the REAL message:

EVERYTHING THEY WANT US TO BELIEVE ABOUT FOOD and NUTRITION IS A LIE.

Whether you choose to believe and act on that is your choice and prerogative... And if you wish to "D"ebate this topic, please provide research that is a notch or two above where you're currently focused.

THE object of good health, is NOT to increase Iron, but to enhance its effectiveness!

THE object is to increase the BIOAVAILABILITY of Iron. The ONLY mechanism to do that is Ceruloplasmin (Cp). Look it up... It's an AMAZING protein wirh 1,056 Amino Acids, that "They" NEVER like to talk about! (It has eight (8) Copper Ions in it...)

So we may differ on our perception of Ascorbic Acid, but I strongly encourage you to dig a little deeper... There's much more to this wholefood Vit-C story, unfortunately...

My ONLY interest is to "D"elete them BOTH as supplements (Homone-D and Ascorbic Acid) as they BOTH are POISON to the human body. That may fly in the face of what you want to "believe," but the REAL research is mind-numbingly CLEAR. You might want to "D"ig into the importance of 13 Cis-Retinoic Acid to Iron Regulatory Proteins...

You might THEN reflect on the FACT that Liver Receptor sites are binary, and MUST choose between Vit-A and Hormone-D...

You might THEN reflect on what impact "D"rowning the body in Hypervitaminosis-D might have on rational, normal Iron regulation and metabolism, esp. in the Liver where it matters MOST...

Food for thought...

Unfortunately, there aren't enough hours in the day to serve up all the REAL studies... I've done more than most, IN MY HUMBLE OPINION, and will add some as I have time...

But the purpose of MAG is to be a TOUCHSTONE for the truth, and reveal what's REALLY going on, inside our bodies...

One bit of advice: ASSUME there is a "They" AND ASSUME "They" are lying to you. That's been my M.O. that has ENABLED me and MAG to get to the TRUTH...

This issue of Ascorbic Acid EXCEEDS the "D"isorientation AND "D"isinfomation of Hormone-D by a factor of TEN (10X)... OMg!...

I am frightened by the HIGH I.Q. of some of the folks in the MAG group, yet the HIGH GULLIBILITY of these SAME folks...

It is most "D"epressing that Robert Thompson, MD and I (and others) labor to introduce light on this "D"esigned "D"arkness and are summarily ignored and challenged by "funded research" -- peer-reviewed or not -- is a VERY SAD COMMENTARY ON OUR TIMES...

The level of "D"ementia re THIS VITAMIN is "D"amnable... As Robert Thompson, MD has so eloquently stated, this is NOT a "D"ebate... This is foundational science.

No boxing gloves needed. Just more people need to read the REAL research...

Robert Thompson
I recognize the confusion. I too have two first hand witnesses, one a student in Dr. Pauling's class where he clearly discussed the whole molecule not being ascorbic acid. We do know that he took large doses of ascorbic acid. I do not know where the

disconnect is. It is however way easier to study ascorbic acid and measure its concentration verses the real molecule.
Regardless of belief (not science), the molecular structure of the C molecule and the ascorbic acid molecule are not the same. Modern technology has clearly clarified that. The work of Dr. Driskol at the University of Kansas has clearly shown the biological effects and mechanism of action of ascorbic acid. It is not the same as the intact C molecule.

I know of other physicians who tout large doses of ascorbic acid for their longevity and health. They are basically taking an antibiotic at that high dose that kills bad bacteria and viruses and possibly oxidizes pre-cancer and cancer cells. They will always pay the connective tissue price eventually due to the total lack of the C molecule in their bodies and poor copper utilization.
Do your homework!

I have given references that should help previously, including the PhD thesis of the graduate student at University of Kansas who did the science, showing that ascorbic acid is a drug, not a vitamin, a pro-oxidant, not an anti-oxidant as is the case of the C molecule in it's intact form, with a mechanism of action that generates H_2O_2 peroxide production inside the cell which is responsible for its effects that are not the same as the actual C molecule.

Remember, the C molecule also has ascorbic acid, and is able to perform the action of ascorbic acid in the cell as well as all the other functions of the C molecule. Ascorbic acid is the binding site of the molecule, so it displaces the C molecule from its binding site and the whole molecule is then excreted. This leaves the cells and the physiology of the human without a molecule needed for life that enables every known copper function in human cells and these are profound. Copper is an essential electron donor in the human, the third most important mineral in human physiology (in some accounts). This is not a debate. This is the science simplified.

But we know 1000 mg of AA/day still acts as anti-oxidant from the study below???

http://www.ncbi.nlm.nih.gov/pmc/articles/PMC2631578/

The authors of that study made several leaps to get to that conclusion and saw the oxidative evidence and ignored it. The study was looking at CRP specifically. There are many reasons that ascorbic acid could lower the CRP both direct and indirect. F2- isoprostane being reduced after ascorbic acid is only an observation without a mechanism or only speculation about one.

This is not enough to make the conclusion that ascorbic acid is an anti-oxidant. Sorry, that will not fly. You need to examine Dr, Driskol's work. It is definitive. Please, this is not a debate. I recognize how messed up the literature is about this because these terms are used interchangeably in nearly all the literature, i.e. Vitamin C and ascorbic acid.

Stimulation of some antioxidant enzymes (especially peroxidase) by the oxidant ascorbic acid (which as I have correctly stated induces the formation of H2O2 in the cells) is much more likely the reason for the errant conclusion and the "antioxidant effect." Remember the Haber-Weiss reaction is equally important, both use iron and electron donors (minerals, usually copper, Mg, Mn, and B vitamins) to complete their contributions to metabolism. I love the Haber-Weiss because it was discovered by the student of Dr. Haber. This all goes together.

There is very little published about the whole molecule and how it breaks down. Think of it ascorbate and ascorbic acid as antibiotics. Then, the effects seen above make sense. Figuring out how to derive the C molecule accurate information out of this literature mess is another huge issue.

In general, I would expect the C molecule to do many of the same things attributed to some of the pieces, and of course much more. The copper issues are nearly always related to the C molecule missing from ascorbic acid being taken or given over too long a period of time or just absolute C molecule deficiency from lack of it in our food.

Actually it is ascorbic acid that does the above, not Vitamin C. It may be explained by the antagonistic effect of Zinc on Copper. Also, one would expect the copper to be unutilized due the ascorbic acid.

I think it all makes more sense when we consider the role of copper in the human (huge) and the need for the C molecule to utilize it. I have had many patients who have been anemic their whole life, and have loaded up on iron and continue their ascorbic acid for years and they do not improve. Those who take the whole C molecule with little or no iron, resolve their life long anemia in about 6-8 weeks, forever. Pretty amazing to watch. I am sure there are many more examples.

But, copper is the key. Iron cannot be incorporated into hemoglobin without copper being there first and the C molecule tyrosinase enzyme allowing it or helping it to do so. There is no tyrosinase enzyme in ascorbic acid, sodium ascorbate, or any of the other imposters. This enzyme also will not work outside of the other cofactors and ions in the C molecule, each molecule of which contains 5 copper ions. Pretty amazing stuff. It is hard to understand how we got so far from the truth of the chemistry of this complex molecule.

Remember when it says something is a Reducing agent, that means it is oxidizing (you probably know that). or pro-oxidant . There can be good reasons for that and bad.

I am not sure why the blue disappears, probably it is oxidation (being reduced). Oxidation is a powerful reaction. Remember, it turns iron to rust.

The inhibition of Tyrosinase by ascorbic acid is another conformation of what I have been saying. I am sure there is more.

Cupric is a crystal like nearly perfectly square molecule of copper and 4 oxygen atoms, in a highly charged form (5.3eV). Stacked in a row of four, that would be 21.2eV. That is the basis of copper batteries. It is amazing to think about the potential of this molecule in biochemical terms.

It would seem that the ceruloplasmin molecule packs a punch, charge wise, and caries a highly charged and reactive form of the Cu atom in suitcase of controlled energy. This may be why the C molecule is so complex, i.e. with enzyme factors and cofactors thereby enabling the highly charged Cu atom to be passed into the biochemistry of the human where and when needed in a positive way.

It is also easy to see how the failure of this transfer could lead to uncontrolled oxidation by this highly charged molecule. So absolutely fascinating. Keep digging. You all are amazing. Cupric atoms, who would have guessed. Another key to the "C" puzzle

.

Truth be known, this relentless "D"ebate about AA vs Wholefood Vit-C is beginning to dull my senses.

This is what we've learned:

o   Copper is ESSENTIAL for 300+ enzymes...

o   ONE of those KEY enzymes is "Ascorbate Oxidase," which REQUIRES Copper to work properly...

o   Copper MUST be bound to Ceruloplasmin to work
      effectively -- it's also known as "Ferroxidase" and is
      SUPREMELY important for Iron, as well...

o   Ceruloplasmin has 6 Copper ions -- of which 2-3 are
      Cupric (Robert Thompson, MD -- what's the significance
      of THAT valence?...)

o   Ascorbic Acid DESTROYS the physiological properties
      of Cp, resulting in its LOSS of "blue" (Ceruloplasmin
      MEANS "Blue Plasma"...) and thus its critical function as
      an Anti-Oxidant!

o   Ascorbic Acid DESTROYS Tyrosinase... Hmmmmm...

How can ANYONE seriously "D"iscuss, much less "D"ebate, this
"Science," as Robert Thompson, MD calls it?!?...

As far as I'm concerned, it's high time for this "D"oubt to end
about why Wholefood Vitamin-C molecule is ABSOLUTELY
ESSENTIAL...

Independent MAG-pie
*In continuing with the mechanism by which AA creates H202 and
in consideration of Quinone redox cycling...*
http://www.ncbi.nlm.nih.gov/pubmed/21395522
*"Ascorbate-driven Quinone redox cycling leads to ROS formation
and provoke an oxidative stress reaction" ...*
I came across this info.

http://www.pnas.org/content/80/1/129.full.pdf
*"at pH 2 the dominant products formed from two-electron
reduction of the Quinone's by ascorbic acid are the
corresponding hydroquinone's and dehydroascorbic acid" and
"with increasing pH, the electrochemical measurements were
more difficult to carry out. Problems associated with rapid
oxidation of the hydroquinone's increased with increasing pH"*

"at pH 7.4 the hydroquinone's are likely to be rapidly oxidized to the corresponding Quinone's" This reaction appears to be dependent on low pH as mentioned above and also here –

http://www.ncbi.nlm.nih.gov/pubmed/9210294

"The present study shows that the inhibitory effect of ascorbate rapidly decreases with increasing pH. At pH 7.4 no significant effect was observed, the result suggesting that ascorbate is not a physiological inhibitor of ceruloplasmin" I suppose what this means is that AA itself does not directly inhibit Cp ...
However it is responsible for the hydroquinone that does inhibit Cp (in presence of free iron and low pH). The reaction of hydroquinone and H2O2 in the presence of free iron is described here...

https://books.google.com/books?id=J0zM5kKXj04Candpg=PA97 2andlpg=PA972anddq=hydroquinone%20and%20fenton%20rea ctionandsource=blandots=bAKUm2dvm2andsig=eBRN7zVfvjGQ boDLoJf3M_9Z3mwandhl=enandsa=Xandved=0CGQQ6AEwCW oVChMIIp_Lt- ubxwIVRBeSCh1LZAse#v=onepageandq=hydroquinone%20and %20fenton%20reactionandf=false

Wholefood C: Ascorbic Oxidase

It's VERY important to distinguish between

o   Vit-C (wholefood Vit-C that earned a NOBEL in 1937...) from

o   Vit-C (Ascorbic Acid that is made with GMO Corn and Sulfuric Acid...)

For the life of me, I can't possibly imagine why we're so hopelessly confused about this VITAL AMINE...

And what's ever MORE outrageous is the TOTAL failure of authors -- clinical or lay -- to point out the IMPORTANCE of Ascorbate Oxidase enzyme -- that is tied to Vit-C/Ascorbic Acid -- but that WILL NOT work unless Copper is present...

http://chemwiki.ucdavis.edu/Wikitexts/UC_Davis/UCD_Chem_12 4A%3A_Berben/Ascorbate_Oxidase

So the question for all those who say that AA and Vit-C are the same...

"Where does the REQUISITE Copper for the Ascorbate Oxidase enzyme come from?!?..."

Hmmmmmmmmmmm?!?...

Wholefood C: Nature vs Test Tube

Ah yes, the familiar "Nature vs Test tube" argument... The "Biologist vs Chemist" argument...

Forgive me, but this is soooooo fatiguing to respond to Facebook members on other sites that are in TOTAL denial about human physiology and its UTTER dependence on minerals...

ALL Oxidase enzymes (Ascorbate oxidase, Lysyl Oxidase, Cytochrome c oxidase, Polyphenol oxidase, to name BUT A FEW!) REQUIRE Copper as a critical catalyst... That is a physiological fact. But no, I don't have a Killer citation to prove my point -- in humans.

There are MANY to show you in the Plant world, but there is TOTAL censorship about this in scientific circles. And while you may NOT want to believe "They" are out to get us, there is OVERWHELMING proof to the contrary...

So, we are left with the lingering reality that we, as a Society, are to believe that synthetic Ascorbic Acid -- made with GMO Corn and Hydrochloric Acid -- is FAR BETTER for us, than a naturally designed and preserved vitamin. That's just more proof of "1984!"...

You will NEVER convince these people that there is a difference. They are acting as "chemists" NOT "Biologists!" There IS a difference...

All we're left with are two KEY questions:

1) HOW does Ascorbate Oxidase Enzyme work WITHOUT Copper?!?...

2) What is the physiological impact of Ascorbic Acid on Ceruloplasmin?!?... They will NOT like either question as they haven't a clue!

My advice, STOP this incessant MBR (Mg Burn Rate) trying to "prove" that MTHR NATURE is smarter than BIG Pharma-funded FB groups, supplement companies, scientists, medical and nursing schools, MOST practitioners, etc.

Yes, it is THAT BAD... Shake it off, and take Mo' Maggie!...
For those that want to better understand Vit-C as Albert Szent-Gyorgyi, PhD studied it (Nobel, 1937), go back to the EARLY research of the 1930's-1940's -- it's a very different perspective... (Please be sure to re-read Robert Thompson's earlier comments)

Ascorbate again the Iron protein, Hephaestin, is THE agent to absorb Iron from your diet. It is put to sleep by excess Calcium (think ridiculous amounts of Hormone-D) and activated by Copper -- found ONLY in wholefood Vit-c.

Ascorbic Acid, regardless of its buffering, HAS NO COPPER... In fact, Ascorbic Acid blocks the Ceruloplasmin, only making your Copper deficiency worse.

Wholefood Vit-C or bust!

People with cancer have elevated levels of UNbound Copper AND Anemic levels of Catalase (CAT)...

What's with that?...

o   CAT is the natural, innate enzyme that the body uses to KILL cancer cells... It's a well-proven mechanism as Marsha is pointing out...

o   CAT can ONLY be made when there are sufficient levels of Bound Copper...

o   What's a proven way to prevent Copper from binding to Cp (Ceruloplasmin)?... HIGH doses of Ascorbic Acid!

So HIGH Ascorbic Acid "mimics" the H_2O_2 function of CAT and ensures that 30 other Copper enzymes are kept deficient for LACK of properly bound Copper...

Ascorbic Acid, the perfect stealth agent for dis-ease and metabolic dys-function...

It boggles the mind, eh?!?...

Wholefood C: Defining It

Wholefood Vitamin-C is like those famous Russian dolls...

o   At the center of Vit-C is the Tyrosinase enzyme...

o   At the center of the Tyrosinase enzyme are 4 Copper Ions...

o   At the center of the Copper ions is your ability to REGAIN your health...

It is KEY to any discussion re this Vital-Amine to draw a CLEAR and metabolic distinction between:

o   Wholefood Vitamin-C that has 6 parts, with the Tyrosinase enzyme at its CORE, that has FOUR Copper ions as part of its construction...

from...

o   The ubiquitous, and worthless (in my humble opinion...) Ascorbic Acid -- that is INCORRECTLY LABELED "Vit-C" -- and is made with GMO Corn and Sulfuric Acid

THEY HAVE NOTHING IN COMMON... But confusion reigns supreme because of the relentless reference to BOTH as "Vit-C" in a society that is easily confused by "Labels."

Were I 'king" for a day, that's one of MANY changes I'd make in the wacky world of nutrition...

Regrettably, all is NOT as it seems...

Ascorbic Acid is a very twisted and distorted concept that is "D"esigned to keep us off balance.

There is NO one article to prove this point, although this one states it very clearly on pages 1057S-1058S:

http://ajcn.nutrition.org/content/67/5/1054S.full.pdf

That is a VERY esoteric article but is does state the TRUTH of Ascorbic Acid -- it causes a depletion of Ceruloplasmin, which is a BIG deal...

And no, the products will NOT say whether they contain Copper -- there is abject censorship about the importance of the mineral... It's complicated and twisted, but it's very real...

Sorry...

Zinc: Factors to Consider

Magnesium's role in the body is to regulate the levels of thousands of minerals, vitamins, enzymes, hormones, neurotransmitters, and genes... Zinc and Maggie are a powerful duo that play a key role in many, many, many activities.

It's important to know that Cortisol is your friend and when it's low, it's likely that you've got too little Potassium, brought on by Adrenal Fatigue that becomes Adrenal Suppression that causes a systemic loss of Sodium and Potassium. And excess Calcium, Copper and Hormone-D work wonders to keep the Potassium in a state of apathy...

It's a very dynamic process, and while hard to believe, is kept in balance and in motion when the body is allowed to keep its Magnesium status at optimal levels... It truly is the "Conductor of the Cell's Orchestra of Minerals..."

The taste bud receptors in our mouth are highly sensitive to Zinc. That's why the Zinc Challenge or Zinc Tally as it is also known, is so helpful. As Meredith notes, it's more anecdotal than empirical, but it's indicative of where your Zinc levels are. These are the broad strokes:

o   Depleted in Zinc: The liquid tastes like water

o   Zinc is returning: The liquid tastes like Cotton Balls for a moment after you swallow...

o   Zinc is really returning: The liquid tastes like Cotton Balls right away...

o   Zinc is Back to Snuff: The liquid tastes like kissing a metal pipe, just as Meredith's husband experienced...

And if you suspect, or KNOW, that you are LOW in Zinc, that's a sure indicator that you are HIGH in unbound Copper that is quite disruptive to the body's optimal metabolism...

Always best to assess this more definitively via HTMA or blood tests, as you have the time or interest in fully addressing these mineral needs...

I have learned to give a wide berth to most supplements that are largely synthetic, as opposed to food concentrates... I'm old fashioned that way... And yes, I do recommend selected "synthetic" Mg supplements...

Why?

Because I know they work and we need the infusion to offset the multi-generational deficiency that has compromised society for the last 100 years!

I don't know for a fact that it's synthetic, but it's got enough syllables to suggest that it does... and I could be widely mistaken, so forgive me if I am...

It is the fact that as a society, we are "Stressed!" to the gills, our Adrenals are the size of pinheads, which then sets the stage for the Adrenals becoming "magnets" for Copper, and the levels of excess, unbound Copper is rising daily from:

o   CuSO4 being put in our water system...

o   CuSO4 being sprayed on ALL our commercial produce...

o   Copper being added to pesticides for Wheat and Beets...

o   Copper being added to Anti-biotics...

o   CuSO4 being added to swimming pools as an anti-fungal...

o   Copper being added to cosmetics...

o   Copper pipes or PVC (which have CuSO4) being the ONLY way water gets into our homes...

o   Copper being a key ingredient in Soy, which is everywhere...

o   Lack of Zinc because folks are being encouraged to "go green," and become vegetarian, which is depleting our bodies of this critical mineral that balances out the Copper...

It's all about balance... and having sufficient energy (Mg-ATP) to properly bind Copper to its target protein, Ceruloplasmin...
Zinc is one of the 15 minerals that is routinely measured on the HTMA.

Also, know that histamine response is HIGHLY dependent on the status of Magnesium and Copper in the body. When there is excess, unbound Copper, it causes an increase of Histaminase, a key enzyme to break down Histamines... And when that gets elevated, it CAUSES a decrease in Histamine systemically... This is well described here:

http://www.tvernonlac.com/copper-toxicity.html

There is a paragraph entitled "Histamine and Methyl" that goes into this dynamic...

Vegan diets are wonderful for detox... It is NOT a sustainable source of nutrients for long term use. Some great suggestions above... (as usual...)

Has this individual done any mineral testing?...

o   Focused: Mag RBC+Copper+Iron Blood Test
o   Complete: HTMA

That would be a great starting point. Several sites that I went to talked about "Alkalizing (Bicarb) liquids" -- Mag Bicarb would be a natural for this and there are recipes in the files for making this.

And yes, the issue with the "animal products" is that she's a "Stress! Cadet," has lost his/her Zinc, and has then lost their HCL which makes the breakdown of more complex sources of food difficult to breakdown...

Also, the Proteases (digestive enzymes that breakdown proteins) are activated by Magnesium...

The MAG-ic KEY to solving the Cu/Zn dynamic and the increased production of Ceruloplasmin (Cp)!

METABOLIC FACTORS

Adrenals

"Burned out" Adrenals are glands missing minerals...

The recognized HTMA mineral ratio for Adrenals is Na/Mg...

The goal of the Adrenal cocktail is to infuse minerals (Sea Salt and Potassium) in a TRUE Vit-C medium that enriches and restores these over-used parts of our anatomy due to our hyper-sympathetic lifestyles. The classic times for the Adrenals to "get tired" are 10am and 3pm...

As a species, we are designed to get up with the Sun, and retire with the Sun. Edison "D"estroyed our natural rhythm and society has suffered mightily ever since!...

Ahhhh, healing the Adrenals...

The three topics that are verboten in conventional medicine:

o   Magnesium deficiency (if they ever even mention Mg...)

o   Copper Toxicity (except as "Wilson's Disease...)

o   Adrenal Fatigue (they ONLY treat Thyroid -- never Adrenals!)

The interplay between those three issues is the key to understanding how to heal the "Stress!" Gland...

First, you need to understand that the Adrenals are RULED by the mineral ratio of Sodium/Magnesium (Na/Mg).

Yes, they make Cortisol (AND 49+ OTHER HORMONES from Cholesterol, mind you...), but their function is dictated by the balance of Na/Mg. You will NEVER heal the Adrenals giving the body synthetic Cortisol. NOT EVER.

That said, there are many whose mineral status is soooo challenged, that they must get that kind of support -- but it is merely a crutch and NOT a solution. You must restore mineral status in the body, and prior to that, you must KNOW mineral status in the body.

Serum blood tests are worthless, as serum is a transport medium OUTSIDE the cell. You NEVER check the Kitchen wall thermometer to assess the OVEN Temp do you?!? No, me neither.

So, if you're spooked by the HTMA, you can spend a fortune and get RBC measurements of Mg, Na, and K (Potassium) and see how balanced or imbalanced you are.

And if you're focusing on "Cortisol Rhythm" testing, all that tells you is that you're "Stressed Out!" and your Rhythm is out of whack -- because of a lack of Maggie... as it is key to recycling Cortisol BACK to its STORAGE form (Cortisone) and regulating the Circadian Rhythm that is SO IMPORTANT for Cortisol production and release over a 24-hr period. Again, it's key to know your Mg status, as noted above...

So, what helps restore Adrenals?:

o   Proper understanding of your mineral status

o   Proper understanding and management of your MBR (Mg Burn Rate) – gotta get your "Stressors!" under control...

o   Broad-based mineral support (mineral drops in H2O,mineral rich diet, etc.)

o   Restoring Mg status in the body (use the "full court" press!)

o   Adaptogen(s): Ashwaganda, Rhodiola, Ginseng, holy basil, Licorice, etc.

o   B-Vitamins from MTHR NATURE (Bee Pollen, rice bran, Beef-liver) (esp. B6)

o   Wholefood Vit-C Complex -- NOT Ascorbic Acid!

o   Many need Liver enzyme support (due to stored Copper and Iron)

o   And everyone's LEAST FAVORITE SUPPLEMENT: SLEEP!!! (9-11 hours/night!)

Please know that this process takes time, but absolutely will respond to nutritional support and sleep. But stemming the Mg leaks in the 2nd bullet point is key...

If you've still got food allergies, if you're still taking Magnesuric Rx meds (most are...),

http://www.ncbi.nlm.nih.gov/pubmed/3822640

If you're still arguing with your spouse, if you're still fighting a low-grade infection, etc. -- your "Stress!" Gland will never get the recovery that it requires, because the Mg leak(s) will prevent recovery.

Also, if you're used to "hard Cardio," give it up! It's only adding to your "Stress!" and will prevent your recovery. A walk around the neighborhood is about all you should be trying to do... And that's very challenging for Adrenal-charged junkies that love to push themselves... which is how you got into this state from the get go, right?...

Sorry for all the blah, blah, blah... Hope that it's helpful...

Unbound Copper, CAUSED by Adrenal Fatigue and an outrageous assault in our food, drugs, and environment, in fact, produces Hydroxyl Radicals (OH) -- AT WILL... These are decidedly toxic to the cell... And what mineral has the most potent effect to neutralize these Radicals?... Why, Maggie, of course!

We can thank a team of Russian scientists who wanted to know the buffering/detoxing effects of the Electrolytes... And Mg won HANDS DOWN!...

Soooooo, too much bio unavailable Copper >> Mg deficiency >> loss of Mg-ATP >> sets the stage for dis-ease and dysfunction... and it works flawlessly and silently... almost like it was planned...

If I were in your body (which I'm not...), I'd wait to get a broader assessment of your minerals -- the very set of information that your doctor is completely ignoring in her/his dictums to take Mo'

Copper!"

I'd tread very carefully down that directive!

I believe the issue is that Copper exists in 2 states in the body...

o   Bio-available: bound to Ceruloplasmin

o   Bio unavailable "free" and NOT bound to Ceruloplasmin

In a "free" state, it is HIGHLY disruptive to the cell, kills Zinc, B6, and binds up Mg++ via the creation of OH (Hydroxyl Radicals) inside the cell.

Plasma Zinc, serum Copper and serum Ceruloplasmin is considered a more definitive measure of what is "bound" and what is "free." Carl Pfeiffer, MD, PhD developed this series of tests 40 years ago...

Regrettably, Copper does exist in BOTH states, and when the Adrenal Glands are weak, they are UNABLE to signal to the Liver to produce Ceruloplasmin (transport protein for Copper), nor are they able to create sufficient energy (Mg-ATP) to bind the "free" Copper (coming from diet, water, BCPs, cosmetics, antibiotics, etc.) to this protein.

Here's a relevant article to explain how central Mg is to this process via the role of Mg-ATP in this process:

https://pure.au.dk/.../ATP7_homology_models_preprint.pdf

This ain't rocket science... Copper Toxicity is CAUSED by

Magnesium deficiency...

The Copper Protocol that we use with clients does both... In fact, there are some who believe a "homeopathic" approach is what is needed: give the body a little bit of what it needs (i.e. bio-available Copper) and it will shed the rest...

We're still researching that approach, but it has merit on some level.
Bio-available Copper includes:

SP Betafood or Livaplex: Liver enzyme support

SP Cataplex C: whole food Vit-C Complex that has Copper enzymes at its core

SP Copper Liver Chelate: when clients have a true physiological need for bio-available Copper

You may do best with Standard Process Adrenotrophin PMG to provide the Adrenals a "diversion" so that they can heal...

When in the process of Adrenal recovery, stressful exercise, besides gentle walking, is ill advised...

Balancing Hormones

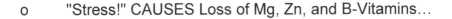

Please follow the bouncing ball..

o   "Stress!" CAUSES Loss of Mg, Zn, and B-Vitamins...

o   When "Stress!" is chronic, the "Stress!" Hormones build, CAUSING the Liver to STOP making Ceruloplasmin (Cp), which changes Copper and Iron status...

o   The greatest source of "Stress!" are the feelings of "helplessness" and "hopelessness..." (Rick Malter, PhD)

o   The enzyme to MAKE Progesterone requires Mg & B6...

o   The enzyme to MAKE Estrogen requires Copper...

o   The mineral that KEEPS Zinc and Copper in proper balance is Mg, with the assistance of B6... (Adolph Butenandt, PhD, 1939 Nobel)

o   ALL 4 forms of PMS are CAUSED by Mg and B6 deficiencies... (Guy Abraham, MD, FACOG)

o   Where a lot of women get into trouble is that their doctor NEVER told them that Birth Control Pills CAUSE Mg deficiency and a build-up of excess, unbound Copper...

o   Also, unbound Copper is VERY toxic due to its oxidative potency to MAKE OH radicals; AND the lack of bound Cu undermines the ability to make Anti-Oxidant enzymes (SOD, CAT, GSH)...

o   Estrogen is MTHR NATURE'S back-up "anti-oxidant" when sufficient Cp can NOT be made... Excess, unbound Cu will facilitate an increase in Estrogen...

o   In my world, the MINERAL comes first!... Yes, there are Xenoestrogens in the environment, but a Copper build-up is FOLLOWED by excess Estrogen -- NOT the other way around...

o   A "popular" bad guy to "cause" loss of Zn and B6 is Pyroluria...

o   Truth be known, Krypto pyrroles occur when insufficient, bound Copper is present to make Haemoglobin -- it is an ENTIRELY Cu-dependent process... Again, increased Oxidative "Stress!" contributes mightily to this issue...

o   Another pervasive toxin that disrupts Mg, Zn, and Cu status is Mercury Toxicity...

As for the DAO elevation during pregnancy, I did not know specifically about that, but it must be in response to Histamines...

But both enzymes to breakdown Histamines, DAO and HNMT, require Mg, Usable Cu and B6 to work properly. That notable increase in DAO would account for why women get so mineral DEPLETED during pregnancy...

That the dynamics of Copper dysregulation are much harder on women... but many of those reasons is the TOTAL LACK OF AWARENESS that "Stress!" CAUSES mineral loss... as noted... Hope that helps you with my perspective on this particular issue...

o   "Is it the Maggie?" -- It is well known that "Stress!" causes hair loss... What's a great way to LOWER "Stress!"?... Take Mo' Maggie!

o   "Is it the Iron?" -- What makes Iron "bioavailable" in the body is usable Copper?... And what makes Copper usable is being attached to Ceruloplasmin (Cp)... And what keep Cp production optimal?... LOW levels of ACTH brought to us by optimal levels of Maggie...

o   "Is your Ferritin better?" -- It is well established in the literature that Copper is a critical factor for optimal Ferritin...

(Just recently I read that it is optimal levels of Cp that ensure optimal levels of Ferritin...)

o   "Maybe your Progesterone?" -- Once again, it's important to understand that Progesterone is ONLY as good as Zinc levels and they are optimal when Copper is NOT in flood stage and Zinc is retained when we're NOT "Stressed Out!"...

o   "Balancing Hormones?" -- It's worth noting that Adolf Butenandt, PhD, the 1939 Nobel laureate for isolating the FIRST human hormones stated later in his career, that the

GREATEST cause of "hormone imbalance" was an imbalance of Calcium and Magnesium...

To the point, there are multiple factors that are associated with Hair Loss and Hair Recovery, but at the end of the trail, it is a common set of mineral factors that dictate optimal metabolism and hair health... not the least of which is our "sponsor," Maggie! There are three Amigos that hang together in the body: Calcium, Copper and Estrogen.

Women who are Estrogen dominant are almost always dealing with excess Calcium and excess, unbound Copper. And until you address ALL 3 legs of the triangle, you'll never resolve their negative impact in the body...

It requires healing the Adrenal Glands FIRST and restoring Mg status as the Calcium: Magnesium balance is what determines the balance of the Hormones.

Despite the relentless programming to the contrary, Hormones do NOT rule minerals... Minerals dictate Hormone status. The key is to have a broad and complete understanding of their actions and interactions...

It's all about restoring balance inside the cell...
The entire cascade of Hormones from Cholesterol >> Pregnenalone >> Steroid "Stress!" Hormones OR Steroid Sex Hormones is regulated by the Cytochrome P-450 family of enzymes -- these are ALL activated by Mg and usable Copper plays a key role, as well!

What the body must do, depending on the level of "Stressors!" is determine which side of the fence or what blend of the two sides that it can produce...

So, at the end of the day, the amount of Mg will dictate your hormone status and balance...

Chronic Fatigue Syndrome

What would be the minerals involved in this enzyme's inability to perform for so many of us with FMS and CFIDS? "Abnormalities of AMPK Activation and Glucose Uptake in Cultured Skeletal Muscle Cells from Individuals with Chronic Fatigue Syndrome".

http://www.wellnessresources.com/health/articles/master_enzyme_switch_deactivated_in_chronic_fatigue_syndrome_and_fibromyalg/

CFS is the wicked intersection of Mg deficiency and Cu dysregulation:

o   The Copper angle:
       http://www.ncbi.nlm.nih.gov/pubmed/18339363

o   The impact on Iron due to bioUNavailable Copper:
       http://www.ncbi.nlm.nih.gov/pubmed/23171474

o   The Magnesium angle to CFS:
       http://web.mit.edu/london/wwwithmagnesium.html

o   Magnesium's role in glucose metabolism...
       http://care.diabetesjournals.org/content/28/5/1175.full

By the way, I could do this ALL day long on just this one issue that plagues millions…

The parallels to hundreds of other chronic conditions should make our minds NUMB that the answer is SOOOO clear, but yet so far...

Here's the TROT:

o   FORGET everything you've read or been told about CFS...

o   Get a comprehensive assessment of your mineral status...(HTMA and Mineral Blood Panels)

o   Work with a nutritional practitioner that understands that the body is RUN by enzymes that ONLY work when MINERALS are present...

o   Follow their recommendations on what to do, and what NOT to do re balancing and restoring your minerals...

o   Do NOT, I repeat, do NOT try to play both sides against the middle -- natural and allopathetic processes do NOT mix, unfortunately...

You have CFS BECAUSE you have mineral dysregulation with Mg, Cu and Iron. Period.

I love Stephen T. Sinatra, MD, FACC's "Metabolic Cardiology," but there are 125 places in that book where he elected to NOT mention Mg or Mg deficiency as the "metabolic catalyst" for proper energy in the heart, as well as the body!

Please take 15 min to read this classic article about how central ATP is to good health and how CENTRAL Mg is to making Mg-

ATP!

http://www.mgwater.com/gafibro.shtml

If you eat REAL food, especially good, clean, grass-fed, hormone-free, red meat, you will get the Carnitine, CoQ10 and D-Ribose... Dr. Sinatra "forgot" to mention THAT, too!

Please get a Mag RBC test asap, so you know how big a climb you have to restore normal metabolic function. Please know that our our metabolism is designed to produce lots of Mg-ATP when were not minerally depleted, as sooooo many are these days...

You do NOT have a "disease!" You have mineral and ATP co-factor deficiencies... BIG difference...

Please know that the MOST POWERFUL SOURCE FOR CREATING EXCESS UNUSABLE COPPER IS WEAK ADRENALS...

A body that is challenged by "Stress!" loses Mg, Zinc and B-Vitamins... This then sets the stage for weakened energy production and weakened protein metabolism which prevents the creation of the key protein, Ceruloplasmin, which is essential to bind Copper and make Iron usable throughout the body. When that happens, excess, unbound Copper builds and the impact is pervasive in the body...

Copper and Glyphosate

http://pubs.acs.org/doi/abs/10.1021/jf00126a010

There is NO more perfect way to bind up Copper in the soil, the plants or the humans...

Glyphosate is BOTH a mineral chelator and an antibiotic which means that it CAUSES Copper dysregulation, as ALL anti-biotics do...

And the reason that we take anti-biotics -- unlike our Ancestors that were Mineral sufficient -- is that LOW Copper >> LOW CuZnSOD >> LOW Macrophage BURST >> HIGH bacteria and infection...

MTHR NATURE'S way for human to CONTROL Bacterial infections are with our innate capacity to produce and USE CuZnSOD to KILL the pathogens BEFORE they can take hold of our system...

That concept is beautifully described and explained in Andre Voisin's book: "Soil, Grass and Cancer" -- the need for Copper is ESSENTIAL to PREVENT Cancer... (No, that was NOT a typo..)

Superoxide Dismutase... It converts the "superoxide free radical" into hydrogen peroxide.... Which then must dealt with by either Catalase of Glutathione to neutralize that H2O2 into H2O...

The synthesis of Glutathione involves two key steps, both of which require Mg-ATP... Those who are "Stressed-out!" are a tad

137

short on their Maggie... Also, the production of ATP requires Zinc AND the recycling of Glutathione (GSH <> GSSG) requires Glutathione Reductase which is Copper dependent...

I'm just beginning to set my sights on MT and what I wonder is whether it plays a similar role for Zinc that Cp plays for Copper... Is there a "usable" and "unusable" capacity for Zinc?... It boggles the mind!!!

Thus, Mercury is the perfectly flawless xenobiotic agent to CAUSE a destruction of both energy pathways, and anti-oxidant defense enzymes...

Not bad.

I can see why Charlie Brown, JD has been struggling for a decade to get this "Mercury Free" Treaty passed on this Planet..

http://www.toxicteeth.org/home.aspx

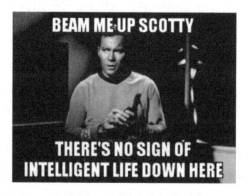

"Beam me up, Scottie!... There appear to be NO signs of intelligent life on this Planet!..."

Copper and Our Thyroid

Copper and thyroid issues imply Copper dysregulation... Either, or BOTH can apply:

o   Lack of bioavailable Copper–to make the Iron bioavailable fires up the Thyroid Peroxidase enzyme: "iodide (I−) is oxidized to iodine (I_0) by the enzyme TPO, called thyroid peroxidase..." THAT CAN ONLY HAPPEN WHEN COPPER IS BIOAVAILABLE…

o   Flip-side: Too much bioUNavailable Copper will BLOCK the Selenoenzyme that cleaves one Iodine off T4 to make T3...Yes, there is a wicked backside to Unbound Copper…

http://www.ncbi.nlm.nih.gov/pubmed/8896290

This is a MUCH more compelling and definitive study done re the impact of Copper deficiency on Thyroid function:

http://naldc.nal.usda.gov/naldc/download.xhtml?id=44230

I've got a call into Dr. Lukaski to learn a bit more and see what other pearls are hidden in the treasure trove of the Human Nutrition Research Center…

That article is a SHOW-STOPPER…

Again, if people will take the time to read it…

If people will take the time to reflect on what it's REALLY saying…

If people will take the time to CHANGE their habitual beliefs and patterns of lifestyle activity…

If people will learn how to IMPROVE their RESPONSE to "Stress!"…

OMg!…

What am I saying?!?…

That's WAAAAAAAY too much to expect!!!

Ceruloplasmin (Cp): What is it?

Transferrin, yet another Copper-dependent protein, does transport Iron, but what MAKES Iron USABLE in the body is Ceruloplasmin. That Cp protein is ALSO called Ferroxidase I by Iron researchers and is the EXACT same protein...

Also, what I've cobbled together is 18 different steps to ensure optimal Ceruloplasmin production in the body: 10 things to STOP DOING, and 10 things to START DOING...

We are what we are routinely told to do by our Mineral Denialist "D"rug pushers...

*** *Please refer to Building Ceruloplasmin*

Very often in the literature, they'll refer to enzymes as proteins... And in the early research on Copper and Ceruloplasmin it is clearly identified as an enzyme...

As for the comment re the "accuracy" of Cp as an indicator of "bound" and "unbound" Copper, I am using this marker X 3 to indicate the # of "units of usable Copper..." It's most helpful in that regard... I shoot to have clients attain a "usable copper" status of 100+, which implies Cp of 35+ (functional Range is 25-40mg/dL)

Ceruloplasmin (Cp): How to Make It

When Copper is NOT attached to its protein partner, Ceruloplasmin (Cp), it is legendary for KILLING:

o   Magnesium...

o   Zinc...

o   B-Vitamins...

Rogue bio unavailable Copper is NOT your friend. But I take a different spin than most -- I focus on RESTORING the production of Cp -- NOT KILLING THE COPPER...

My focus is NOW squarely on supporting the Liver's production of Ceruloplasmin (Cp) with the intent being to make the Copper productive. The vast majority of folks that I've worked with have anemic levels of Cp -- <25mg/dL, many <20...

This is my game plan:

1) **STOP** Hormone-D ONLY Supplements, that KILL Vitamin-A, given that Vitamin-A is a critical precursor to Cp production...

2) **STOP** Calcium supplements that BLOCKS Copper absorption, given that Copper is needed to make Cp and BLOCKS Maggie absorption, as well...

3) **STOP** Iron supplements to solve "Iron Anemia," given that in the research literature it is VERY CLEAR that this is a

clinical sign of Copper deficiency, and excess supplemental Iron SHUTS DOWN Copper metabolism

4) **STOP** Ascorbic Acid as it CAUSES Copper to separate from Cp and destroys the enzyme Tyrosinase…

5) **STOP** HFCS and Synthetic Sugars excess Fruit (Fructose), in your diet as it is perfectly designed to LOWER Liver Copper and ELEVATE Liver Iron

6) **STOP** LOW Fat Diet, fat is essential for proper Copper absorption.

7) **STOP** Using Industrialized, "Heart Healthy" Oils!

8) **STOP** Using products with Fluoride *toothpaste, bottled water, etc)

9) **STOP** Taking Multi & Prenatals, they have the first 4 items

10) **START** Mg supplements to lower ACTH (5mg per lb/ 10mg per kilo of body weight)

11) **START** Cod Liver Oil (1 Tbsp of Nordic Naturals - Artic, or Rosita's)

12) **START** Wholefood Vit-C (500-800 mgs/day)

13) **START** Boron -- 1-3 mgs/day (aids in Synthesis of Cp) to deliver the cofactors, Tyrosinase and Copper ions that the Liver needs for Cp…

14) **START** Boron – Boron (no more than 3mg/day) as it, too, plays a role in Cp production, but I'm a bit fuzzy on exactly what it is, but know that 98% of all HTMA clients are LOW in Boron…

15) **START** B2 (Riboflavin) -- Key for Cu/Fe regulation in Liver, B-Vitamins to be sure to get B2 (Riboflavin) and B7 (Biotin) which are important to Liver function, and especially the roles of Iron and Copper...

16) **START** Biotin (B8) – Key for Cu/Fe regulation in the Liver

17) **START** Ancestral Diet (HIGH Fat/Protein/LOWCarb)

18) **START** Mo' Maggie to stem the rise of ACTH which KILLS Cp production in the Liver...

19) **START** Taurine to support Copper metabolism in the Liver.

20) **START** Iodine as it is critical in the production of Cp, given that it is key to the Iodinization of critical Amino Acids that make Cp...

This last step is a major step and requires BOTH optimal RBC Selenium and RBC Magnesium before delving into this process...

https://www.facebook.com/groups/MagnesiumAdvocacy/permalink/832711093463628/

https://www.facebook.com/groups/MagnesiumAdvocacy/833149540086450/?hc_location=ufi

To be bio-available, Copper MUST be bound to its transport protein, Ceruloplasmin (Cp). I call it the Chaperone, given the scientific symbol "Cp"...

So, Copper **with** the Chaperone is **GOOD**...

And Copper **without** the Chaperone is **BAD**...

Copper, without that Chaperone is considered BAD as this protein produces a critical enzyme needed to PREVENT iron from being a major source of oxidation (aka, "rust!") in the body and in the cells...

Cp is a major anti-oxidant...

So is Estrogen! Who knew?...

So the body will use that hormone as a "back-up plan" to provide an anti-oxidant for this Metal. The key to Boron is that it plays a critical role in enhancing Liver function, and works with Vitamin-B2 to keep Copper and Iron in proper balance... It also has a known effect in increasing the production of The Chaperone, which is KEY to improving Copper bio-availability in the body..."

Elevated Ceruloplasmin (Cp) is linked with pregnancy, birth control pills, infection and increased Inflammation. Cp is referred to as an "acute phase protein" that responds to an inflammatory assault. And what triggers inflammation is Mg deficiency (Weglicki and Phillips, 1992; Raysigguier, 1993)

I'm not sure what' tripped your wire, but that's the likely cause of your Cp elevation. Knowing your overall mineral profile would be KEY to better understanding these dynamic's...

Ceruloplasmin (Cp): Increasing Production

The principle sites of Cp production are in the Liver and the Brain...

Please note, Allopatheic Medicine that IS Affagato, is training us -- like Circus Bears -- to view this life-enhancing anti-oxidant enzyme as a "toxin" and to link it with the inflammatory process...

It's the perfect way to create "Booga-Wooga" reactions by the public and the practitioners that keep them in the "D"ark with their infantile understanding of how the body REALLY works... Based on my assessment over the last 4 decades...

o   You gotta be REALLY smart to get into medical school...

o   You gotta be REALLY compliant to get out of medical school...

o   You gotta be REALLY numb to the reality that your adrenal medication is NOT working to succeed in practice...

Hormones and Magnesium

http://www.ncbi.nlm.nih.gov/pubmed/3840173

It would be worth your purchasing this article Robert K. Rude, MD has the most enlightened, accurate and Mg-truth-based perspective on Hormones and Maggie...

Please note the date on this article...

Forgive me, I've not had a chance to review this series of studies, but let me share some Mineral-based observations:

o   Hormones, like "D" -- IT IS NOT A VITAMIN! -- REQUIRE action. They are very powerful chemicals designed to change/protect mineral status...

o   Pump in outrageous amount of unopposed Hormone-D and the body is FORCED to flip the Storage form of the Hormone to its ACTIVE FORM -- which REQUIRES Mg!

o   Deng et al 2013 CLEARLY demonstrates the Mg DRAIN CAUSED by Hormone-D metabolism... There is NOTHING subtle about it...
http://www.biomedical.com/1741-7015/11/187

o   Furthermore, Inflammation is CAUSED by Mg deficiency (Weglicki and Phillips, AmJrlPhysiol, 1992). This foundational, metabolic FACT is summarily IGNORED worldwide ... WHY? It destroys the Biz Model of BIG Pharma..

o   What I am also seeking to sync with is the fact that Hormone-D will disrupt Retinol (Vit-A), a critical precursor to Cp, thereby rendering Copper unusable, which CAUSES an increase in Oxidative Stress as the Anti-Oxidant enzymes (SOD, CAT, and GSH) are dependent on bioavailable Copper! (Am I the ONLY MAG-pie that sees that supplemental "D" is the PERFECT stealth agent to CAUSE Inflammation AND Oxidative Stress?!?...)

So, I would encourage you to re-read these articles with an understanding of those mineral and metabolic premises... They read VERY differently when you realize that the MINERAL LOSS is the "D"og -- and NOT "D"tail...

Hypertension And Adrenals

The reason why MOST Cinnamon does NOT work is that it is sawdust, sprayed with oil... You get what you pay for... Cinnamon from Viet Nam is an entirely different spice...

Again, hypertension is invariably due to Electrolyte imbalance... different strategies will work, but at the core is the need to restore Mg, and correct excess Calcium and too little Sodium (yes, that is NOT a typo...) Very often, excess unmanaged Iron is a factor, as well.

I'm assuming that if it says organic, it should be OK... But as they say in the desert: "Trust Allah, but tie up your camel..."

I'd call just to verify...

Also, it is likely that your Hypertension stems from excess, unbound Copper that was revealed in your HTMA and is likely being stored in your Kidneys. It intensifies the Sympathetic Response, and can cause an elevation of blood pressure, as Copper is quite toxic to Mg, and Potassium and elevates Sodium, which is a recipe for Hypertension...
Ways to create "excess, unbound Copper":

o   FASTEST WAY: Adrenal fatigue!

o   Cut back on meat, which is loaded with Zinc, its mineral antagonist!

o   Focus on these foods:

- eat Commercial (NOT Organic) produce -- it's sprayed with CuSO4 (an anti-fungal agent...)
- Soy anything...
- Avocados...
- Nuts and Seeds...
- Chocolate (not Cacao...)

o   Use Birth Control Pills or a Copper IUD

o   Copper pipes bring H2O into the home...

o   Municipal water has CuSO4 as an "anti-fungal"

o   Swimming pools use CuSO4 as well...

o   Cosmetics have lots of Copper

o   Anti-biotics often have Copper in them...

What's key is to have healthy Adrenal Glands (proper balance of Sodium and Magnesium) to ensure ability to make Ceruloplasmin which Copper needs to be bound to... And plenty of Mg-ATP which requires healthy Adrenals, as well...

Those are just the Headlines...
Please note, the secret to Dr. Bat's "water therapy" is the minerals THAT MOST H2O IS MISSING...

o   We are 72% H2O...

o   We are 28% Minerals...

o   Mg is "hydrophilic"... (LOVES Water...)

o   Ca is "hydrophobic"... (HATES Water...)

Yes, it's that basic...
"Distilled" water is "hungry" water... what is it hungry for?
Minerals! And that's a fact...

We regularly filter our well water and then re-mineralize it with
minerals from either The Great Salt Lake (Anderson's CMD) or
off the coast of Australia (www.SeaMineral.com)

When we're "thirsty," the body is seeking two elements:

o H_2O; and
o   The 80+ minerals that our Ancestors took for granted,

and we have to fight for because of the toxic nature of "municipal
sanitation" and global water bottling corporations...

Nestle is the Monsanto of water, by the way...

The Big "D"iscussion

Forgive me, but I'm gonna be an incessant bore about this issue...

If you are basing your "D"ecision to take copious amounts on of D-only supplements based on a 25(OH) blood test...

Please step back and ask yourself 4 important questions:

1)   What is my Mag RBC?...

2)   Is my daily intake of Cholesterol, Mg and Sun adequate, to support healthy metabolism?...

3)   How does my doctor earn a living? (When I'm healthy or when I'm sick!...)

4)   What is the tgist of the research on Hormone-D REALLY saying that is being compiled in the MAG FB Group Photo File?!?

Hmmmmmm?!?...

Has anyone taken the time to read any of the articles that are posted here?

https://www.facebook.com/photo.php?fbid=600557466658064andset=oa.574059815995425andtype=3andtheater

Please take a moment and familiarize yourself with the research on this HORMONE...

It is NOT a vitamin you're dealing with here...

It's very seductive and very easy to take, but do you really KNOW what mineral impact it is having INSIDE your body?

NO, you don't and neither does your doctor -- despite the "glowing" accolades that are heralded from the research, and the endless articles from the internet.

Take a step back and calmly study what the research is REALLY saying...

Let me qualify...

Yes, I am quite strident about not getting "D"eceived by the currently popular supplement routines... But what's laced in my overtures are two points:

1)   Please read some objective research -- outside the U.S. -- that is clearly calling this "D"ietary "D"ictum into question...

       and

2)   Please get your minerals tested (HTMA) and find out what impact this HORMONE is really having inside your body...(25(OH) and 1,36(OH) blood test)...

And why do folks think they feel "better" on this routine?... I don't truly know, I've got some theories, and am researching that regularly... At this point, me thinks it's more "placebo" than "purposeful." More than likely the level of calcium rises, due to increased levels of calcitriol, that is causing "metabolic numbness."

I appreciate the points that you are seeking to make "two miles up..." re the rich diversity of what we need to exist on this Blue Marble hurling through space...

Please take 10 minutes and read this classic article sloooowly:

http://www.mgwater.com/gacontro.shtml

Please don't assume that you KNOW what Dr. Abraham is talking about. Yes, Vit-D is an important part of our intake, but not in isolation, as you aptly note.

What's vitally important is to know that our Ancestors lived in a Magnesium-rich environment, which was very "Calcium-poor." And Vit-D played a key role IN THAT ENVIRONMENT.

Tragically, our environment changed DRAMATICALLY ~1900 with the advent of "modern" farming and food processing to create a Calcium-RICH environment THAT IS NOW INCREASINGLY DEVOID OF MAGNESIUM. And those are the facts.

What's key here is to understand HOW our bodies are designed to make Hormone-D naturally, when fed good clean fats (which supply Vit-A and Cholesterol, the precursor to Hormone-D!), rich sources of Magnesium and yes, being regularly kissed by the Sun.

So, there is a major metabolic difference by the way the

Hormone-D we create naturally, and the toxic swill folks are swigging daily -- completely oblivious to the mineral gyrations that it creates in the human body lacking Vit-A and Magnesium, which most suffer from. If you haven't studied hair tissue mineral analyses, like I and my HTMA colleagues have, you lack the rich mineral profile context to understand what I'm talking about.

The point that almost ALL miss in the studies is that in MOST "Vit-D Research studies" they measure 25(OH)D (Calcidiol -- storage form) in the blood, and THEN FOR THE EXPERIMENT, ADMINISTER 1,25(OH)2 (Calcitriol -- Active form).

At the carnival and the used car lots, we call that "BAIT AND SWITCH!" And it's done all the time in these so-called "pure" research studies as the public, and apparently the practitioners, are clueless that it exists in different forms... There is a MAJOR metabolic difference between a Hormone's "storage" and "active" states...

All is NOT as it seems and I welcome you to study this aspect of "D"ietary "D"ictumland very carefully as it is the most confusing and confounding of all aspects of nutrition.

I welcome your questions and push back, but PLEASE DON'T SHOOT THE MESSENGER...

Is Vitamin D the same thing as Vitamin D3?
Yes, they are used interchangeably which is where the confusion lies...

o   Pre-HORMONE = Cholecalciferol
o   Storage form of HORMONE = Calcidiol
o   Active form of HORMONE = Calcitriol

If I were King for a day, I would REQUIRE ANYONE discussing this "D"emonic topic to use the scientific names and NEVER the "D" or "D3"

It creates TOTAL confusion, which apparently what they were seeking to do, and I'm convinced they have accomplished their appointed task...

What I'd advise is that you "lift the hood" on your mineral status, and see where both your Mag RBC is, as well as your overall mineral profile (HTMA).

Without that bedrock information, and basing your Vit-D intake solely on a "flawed" blood test, without knowing your true Mg status, is a very risky thing to do...

I do apologize for your confusion, but I'm dancing as fast as I can to sort out the facts and the truth... something very novel in the world of nutrition...

Here's the link that has the Hormone-D articles...

https://www.facebook.com/photo.php?fbid=600557466658064an dset=oa.574059815995425andtype=3andtheater

At the risk of sounding braggadocious... the information being offered on this MAG Facebook Group is FAR closer to the truth and far more balanced than the vast majority of Internet drivel that gets copied copiously from website to website to website, never bothering to verify whether the "data" contained is at all accurate...

Truth be known...

o   I have never seen God, but do believe in a higher being...

o   I have never seen a Mg ion, but am certain of its supremacy in our body as BOTH mineral foundation and Conductor of the Cell's Mineral Orchestra...and its ability to activate ATP -- the energy of life...

o   I have never seen a Fluoride ion, a Calcium ion, a Copper ion, nor a Hormone-D molecule, etc., but I KNOW how toxic each of them is to Mg status...

Until you do the HTMA, you'll have no idea of whether that Vlt-D is doing what that "book" told you it would. Also, please know that "Vit K2" must be phosphorylated and carboxylated before it can do its work -- BOTH steps require Mg-ATP!!!

In my humble opinion, you need Mo' Maggie to make either of those "so called" vitamins work... And if the multi you're taking has Mo Calcium than Maggie, then you're NOT getting the Magnesium you so critically need...

My intent is NOT to confuse... The process to move from K1 >> K2 requires Mg-ATP... But you have two forms of K2 which suggests that they've done the work for you, albeit synthetically.

That said, you should be OK, but I put faaaaaar more stock in the importance of Mg to regulate Calcium status, due to its regulatory role with ALL 3 Hormones that regulate Calcium: Calcitonin, PTH and Hormone-D. I'm not as bullish as most are with K2...

o   Calcium is elevated because Mg is Low...

o   Vit-D is low because Mg is Low...

o   Iron is likely low because the uptake enzyme, hephaestin is dependent on whole Vit-C Complex, which MUST be activated by Mg...

o   B-12 is dependent on a Mg-dependent enzyme to get inside the cell...

ALL four of your "issues" relate to the status of Mg. It's best to start HERE and see where your markers are FOLLOWING a focus on Mg.

And no doubt you're wondering: "So why doesn't my doctor know all this?!?..."

I've got the EXACT SAME question...

Any committed farmer knows that outside of sunshine and rain -- neither of which they can control -- the most important focal point is the pH of the soil, and that is solely regulated by MINERALS!

It's absolutely the same inside our "soil," as well... It's just that no one ever told you how vital and how basic these powerhouse elements are in maintaining the electrical and physiological integrity of the body...

Please know, that any "supplement" that has Calcium + VitD3 will deliver NO Magnesium... And that's a scientific fact!

You are well advised to not promote products that don't promote

Magnesium restoration on this Facebook page...

And it might serve you well to read this article carefully:

www.gotmag.org/the-vitamin-d-controversy/

ALL IS NOT AS IT SEEMS...

Sorry to be the messenger...

Dr. Dai at Vanderbilt University identified the dynamic between Calcium and Magnesium:

o   Excess Calcium to Magnesium BLOCKS Mg   absorption

o   Excess Magnesium to Calcium GUARANTEES Calcium absorption

http://www.ncbi.nlm.nih.gor/pmc/articles/PMC3320715/

Hormone-D (Calcitriol, the Storage form of the Hormone) will ALWAYS be LOW when there is insufficient Mg to activate it, or said another way, the REAL reason why it's low is that the body KNOWS that there is EXCESS Calcium in the blood and that taking any more will cause the Calcium levels to increase.

Despite what you've been trained - - like a Circus Bear - - to believe, Maggie is your friend, and Calcium -- NOT SO MUCH!

Please read this article to gain a clearer understanding of just how toxic "excess Calcium" really is;

http://www.naturalnews.com/038286_magnesium_deficiency...

And as you have further questions because of the counter-cultural nature of this metabolic truth, please ask away...

It turns out that Jean Durlach, MD, a gifted French Mg Researcher, once said to NEVER exceed 2 parts Calcium to 1 part Mg...

Some enterprising soul in BIG Pharma took that "caution" and twisted it into a "LAW" and "Homo Calcificous" has NEVER been the same.

Sea water, which we evolved from, has 3 parts Magnesium and 1 part Calcium...

Current Western diet is estimated to be ~5 parts Calcium and 1 part Magnesium...(Rosanor, 2010)

The rate of Chronic Disease is at Tsunami proportions... fueled in LARGE part to excess Calcium, and from fotification, that is overwhelming the human metabolism...

We all know that Calcium is "good" for strong bones, right?... Well, as a former Hospital guy, I can assure you that Calcium is "good" for STRONG BOTTOM LINES for doctors and hospitals. (Please re-read comment re meteoric rise of chronic disease above.)

ALL IS NOT AS IT SEEMS...

And if you can find a legitimate, bona fide research study that backs up what you say, I'll be delighted to read it and if convinced of their argument, I'll eat crow for you on MAG!

How's that?!?...

Chances are you have very little valid information about your "true" mineral status... Serum measurements are NOT valid, as serum is "extracellular..." RBC measurements are QUITE valid (because they ARE Intracellular), but can get a bit pricey...

HTMA (hair tissue mineral analysis) is QUITE VALID (it's looking at tissue levels), but we are "conditioned" to question ANYTHING that is NOT BLOOD as a shaky source, and that is reinforced by practitioners who have been "TRAINED" to regard HAIR as "pure quackery," which it is NOT.

You have likely read hundreds of articles, and heard from ALL your family, friends, and work buddies, telling you to take Vitamin-D, but what you did NOT know is that they failed to tell you the following:

o   Vitamin-D is a HORMONE...and a very powerful one at that...Despite it's popularity, we as a species are NOT designed to EAT Hormones, but are designed to make them from Cholesterol... Hmmm... (You mean Cholesterol is actually good for my health?!?...)

o   Hormone-D MUST be in balance with Retinol (animal-based) Vitamin-A - - it has been that way since the dawn of time...

VERY FEW tell you that! Chris Masterjohn, PhD is a noted exception and authority here:

http://blog.cholesterol-and-health.com/

o   That the conversion of Cholesterol >> Prehormone-D >>
        Calcidol >> Calcitriol ALL require ENERGY (Mg-
        ATP) and Magnesium... Excess intake of "D" really
        drains your Maggie!

o   That ALL 3 Hormones (Calcitonin, PTH and Hormone-D)
        that dictate levels and Location of Calcium are ALL
        activated by Mg... Imagine that... no one has stressed
        that, have they?...

o   That Vitamin-K, the latest MSM nutrient darling,
        MUST be Carboxylated and Phosphorylated to be
        biologically effective -- fancy words for just another way
        to burn MORE Mg-ATP...

o   That your doctor NEVER suggested you get 3 blood
        tests to accurately assess your need for "D":

        -       Mag RBC (Ref Range: 5.0-7.0mg/dL -- please
                ignore the current Lab Range!)

        -       25(OH)D -- Storage Form (Calcidiol)

        -       1,25(OH)2 D3 -- Active Form (Calcitriol)

If #1 is >6.0mg/dL AND #3 is LOW (just IGNORE #2...), then and
ONLY THEN take a food-based form of Hormone-D, just like
your Ancestors did for thousands of years... Yes, somehow they
survived and you will, too...

o   And yes, Hormone-D, the OLDEST HORMONE ON
        PLANET EARTH, is designed to get Calcium INTO
        the blood (Please note thatVitamin-A gets it into the

Bone...) because the environment was very Mg rich, and Calcium poor and it was that way for millions of years until ~1900 when the Food Processors started to change it...

And excess dietary and supplementary Calcium is NOT your metabolic friend and the research is PROVING THAT IN SPADES... Trust me, there's a reason why managing Calcium (which is Mg's job in the body, by the way...) is "Job #1" at BIG Pharma... Can't rely on a mineral that CANNOT be patented, let's use Synthetic Rx Meds, that CAUSE Mg Loss, and we'll make billions!... (You think I jest, I'm sure...)

So, waaaaaaaay too much blah, blah, blah... but this topic is MY "Job #1" to wake MAG-pies up to the metabolic reality of their body, and beat the drums of sanity in allowing the body to get back to balance...

I'll look forward to the blow-back and questions that this will stimulate...

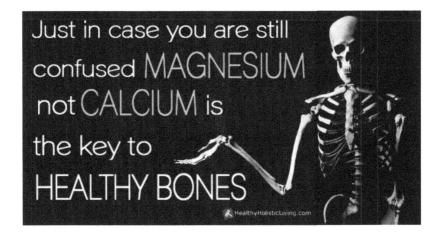

Just in case you are still confused MAGNESIUM not CALCIUM is the key to HEALTHY BONES

Magnesium, NOT Calcium, Is the Key to Healthy Bones
Until now all of us, and probably you too, thought that calcium is the element most needed in order to have a healthy bone structure, right? Well it is very

A good starting place before engaging in Hyper-D supplementing is to get the key tests:

o   Mag RBC

o   1,25(OH)D (Active form of the Hormone-D, Calcitriol)

o   25(OH)D (Storage form of the Hormone-D, Calcidiol)

It is key that you know ALL 3 of these numbers. Yes, Mg is used up in significant levels with "D" supplementation, but what is coming to light is the fact that storage levels and active levels of "D" are two very different beasts. And it is very likely that your Active Hormone-D is elevated and you are NOT aware of that.

I'm not sure of what your neurological condition is, but know that Mg-ATP and Vit-B3, and B6 are vitally important in energy production in the brain (and elsewhere...).

I'd get these tests and have certainty driving your decisions, not clinicians who have NO training in Magnesium metabolism. And how do I know that? They never test for it, they never recommend its use, and they are totally unaware of the fact that 3,751 proteins and over 2,000 enzymes MUST have Mg and/or

Mg-ATP to properly function. Not an insignificant oversight in their medical education... in my humble opinion.

Our Ancestors lived in Northern climates for thousands of generations and compensated for this issue with their diet: free-range eggs, happy bacon, grass-fed Liver, wild-caught deep sea fish, fermented Cod Liver Oil, etc. This is NOT a "new" issue...

There are several key issues with "D" supplementation:

1)   NO ONE ever told you that there are two different tests for "D" status...25(OH) [Storage] and 1,25(OH) [Active]

2)   NO ONE ever told you how important Vit-A is to metabolizing Hormone-D... they are biological antagonists~!

3)   NO ONE ever told your how demanding Hormone-D was on Magnesium status...

4)   NO ONE ever told you how synthetic "sheep skin oil being illuminated by commercial lighting" is...

5)   NO ONE ever told you that food sources for "D" exist, and have existed, to properly balance the need for this Hormone...

6)   NO ONE ever told you that what Active Hormone-D does is ELEVATE Calcium in the blood -- not necessarily to your advantage...

7)   NO ONE ever told you about the impact excess

Hormone-D has on your Potassium status, which is that it CAUSES it to crash...

I do apologize for the angst that this is creating. Sometimes, the truth does hurt...

Please read this excellent article by Chris Masterjohn, PhD, a rising star in the world of nutrition...

http://www.westonaprice.org/.../new-evidence-of-synergy.../

The numbers to achieve balance might surprise you...

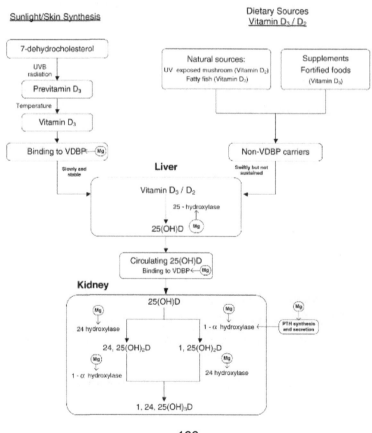

You might go to the Files section and read through some of the articles, especially, the one by Xinqing Deng has a wonderful flow diagram on the role of Mg...(Please find on next page.

http://www.biomedcentral.com/1741-7015/11/187

This is the hidden story that very, very few know about Hormone-D...

The human body is a series of seesaws... There are many, many, many biological partners and antagonists that work to stay in balance and keep us in homeostasis...

The Conductor of that Cellular Orchestra on Minerals is Magnesium... much to the wonderment of the masses and much to the frustration of BIG Pharma...

As we learned all too painfully from the Cholesterol Con job and Heart Disease, "correlation" does NOT mean "causation..."

By the way, please ask yourself, do flies CAUSE garbage?...

Of course not, and the fact that Cholesterol collects in energy-starved heart muscle cells has NO bearing on heart disease, and the same likely holds for Hormone-D and MS. It is likely a relationship of correlation...

Vit "D" Receptors (VDR)

o   VDR is regulated by Magnesium (Mg-ATP)...

o   Under "Stress!" we lose Maggie, and others minerals...

o	VDR bsm is an epi-genetic response to "Stress!"...

o	It's MTHR NATURE'S way of adapting to our insane lifestyles and diets...

(VDR = Vitamin D Receptor... Most, if not all, receptors misbehave when Maggie's missing...)

Preferred brands of CLO that have HIGH ratio of Vit-A:Vit-D (which is KEY!) Are:

o	Nordic Naturals - Artic
o	Rosita's Real Food Extra Virgin CLO

Is there danger of too much Vit-A build up in the liver???

The only danger is believing that MTHR MATURE would allow this to happen despite generations of people ingesting PROPER ratios of these oils in their foods...

We live in a most challenging world, n'est ce pas?...

I recognize that there are flaws in ANY product that we buy. I have come to realize that Nordic Naturals Artic and Rosita's Real Food CLO are likely the two best CLOs -- amidst a sea of marginal sources -- to OFFSET the gross toxication by Storage-D that is compromising health globally.

These are NOT perfect options but, they RIGHT A SERIOUS WRONG that has been perpetrated on an unsuspecting public. It is vital that our Livers have sufficient Retinol to work with.

I don't know what the sources are on Vit. Shoppe and Nature's Bounty, nor do I know what a 15:1 vs 10:1 is...

What I DO KNOW is that the global obsession with D: ALOT is CAUSING a lot of mineral imbalance and metabolic dysfunction...

Your Potassium is tanked and that's going to be key to your full recovery... Low Potassium is VERY stressful on our body, our heart, and out mind...

And what brings it back?...

CLO with a 10:1 dose of Vit-A to Vit-D like that found in Rosita's Real Food CLO or Nordic Naturals - Artic...

OK, here's the deal..

Calcium has NEVER been the problem!... And thus Hormone-D is NOT the priority!

But Vit-A (Retinol, NOT Beta-carotene...) IS KEY, as it is ESSENTIAL to ensure optimal production of Ceruloplasmin (Cp) in the Liver. (Excess Hormone-D SHUTS CP production DOWN!)...

But MTHR NATURE understands the importance of metabolic balance, so 10-parts Vit-A to 1-part Hormone-D is what's required! (Remember, "D" is a Hormone and it takes 10 Retinols to keep it in check!!!)

Brands that "appear" to understand and honour that ratio and its importance are:

o   Rosita's Real Food CLO

o   Nordic Naturals - Artic (NOT the Artic-D!)

If there are others, please bring them to our attention!

"BEFORE jumping on that band-wagon, I would simply ask
anyone to do the following:

o   Please measure these three markers in your blood:

-       Magnesium RBC
-       25(OH)D -- Storage form of Hormone-D (Calcidiol)
-       1,25(OH)2 D3 -- Active form of Hormone-D
        (Calctriol)

If your Mg RBC >6.0mg/dL AND your ACTIVE Hormone-D is
LOW, then, and ONLY then do you need supplementary support.
And if #1 and #3 are BOTH LOW, I would strongly advise you
work on #1 FIRST.

o   Assuming that you've done these ESSENTIAL blood tests
        and have confirmed a true, physiological "need" for "D,"
        please use food-based forms of Hormone-D that have
        graced this Planet for thousands of years.

-       Fermented Cod Liver Oil
-       Grass-fed Liver
-       Free-range Eggs
-       Wild caught, deep-sea fish

Why is that important? You absolutely need balancing sources of
Vitamin-A (Hormone-D's biological antagonist and partner) to

properly support its being used in the body. Yes, Vit-K is helpful, but Vitamin-A is ESSENTIAL and rarely gets the nod.

Now I realize that I'm a total nudge on this issue, but the research is more and more supporting the FACT that hyper-supplementation of synthetic "D" is NOT warranted, nor healthy."

The Calcium Wars... Please read this article that Carolyn Dean, MD, ND and I wrote a couple of years ago:

http://www.naturalnews.com/038286_magnesium_deficiency

And this article by Guy Abraham, MD seals the deal:

http://www.mgwater.com/gacontro.shtml

Last licks, Robert Thompson, MD's book is a must-read and a God-send for those seeking the truth re Calcium vs. Magnesium...

Most people are OBSESSED with their Vit-D levels and are CLUELESS about their Ceruloplasmin (Cp) levels -- and the two are tightly connected! (Only Vit-D supplements KILL Liver Retinol that is a critical precursor to Cp...)

Depending on how LOW the "usable" Copper level is, determines whether I use/don't use Zinc. It is exceptionally powerful in lowering Copper, by how it blocks Copper absorption, which may or may not be advisable -- depending on your actual situation. This process is NOT about "detoxing" Copper...

It IS about "goosing up" more Ceruloplasmin, and I've got ~20 steps to make sure that it happens...

If you've been under notable "Stress!", know that that affects your status of Mg, Zn, B Vitamins, and when the "Stress!" becomes chronic, bioavailable Copper takes a hit due to the lowered production of Cp...

Hope that makes sense... Looking forward to your further questions and assisting you gain balance...

There is NO clinical benefit to having Storage-D above 21, "D"espite the relentless "D"in of articles suggesting it should be over 70, which is UTTER nonsense...

http://www.sciencedaily.com/rele.../2013/05/130501192929.htm

You might want to read this article as well:

http://gotmag.org/vitamin-d-deficiency-mg-deficiency-period/

CONDITIONS

Cardiac Afibrillation (Afib)

AFIB is "Stress!"-induced Mg loss >> electrolyte derangement...

It is NOT a medical disease...

It is metabolic dysfunction from mineral deficiencies (Mg & K)...

You might print out a copy for their cardiologist so he can learn how the Heart really works!...

Please share this document:

http://www.afibbers.org/conference/PCMagnesium.pdf

Research changed in the early '80's under Reagan's tutelage...

 The Fox is now guarding the henhouse and if you think the "contemporary discoveries" are NOT engineered to support the sale of MORE toxic, synthetic, and mineral-depleting Rx meds, then I've got both a bridge and a used BMW I'd love to sell ya!

In two words, your relentless din of veiled support for BIG Pharma is both fatiguing and unwelcome...Is THAT focused enough for you?...

If you have AVN from steroids along with the congested heart failure....

I had the distinct pleaseure of a private conversation with Suzy Cohen, RPh after reading this wonderful and revealing article:

http://www.jigsawhealth.com/blog/drug-muggers-suzy-cohen-magnesium

ALL Classes of Cardiac Rx meds create "Stress!" >> Mg Loss...

The most important book ANYONE with heart issues should read is Stephen T. Sinatra, MD, FACC "Metabolic Cardiology" -- the TRUTH of Mg's role in Cardiac function is clearly spelled out there! There is even a chapter devoted to Mg and it's role on heart health.

The ENTIRE field of Cardiology exists for lack of Mg-ATP -- brought about by "Stress!"-induced loss of Maggie and bioavailable Copper.

Antibiotics

Antibiotics are designed to block Copper... I'm guessing the ones with Fluoride (Floxies...) are especially good at that...

Take away the Copper, and you take away the body's ability to MAKE anti-oxidant enzymes... and when they are missing, the symptoms of IBS, Crohns, Colitis come out of the wood work...

These are NOT medical diseases... They ARE definitive signs of metabolic dysfunction CAUSED by mineral deficiencies...

Please note that Silver BLOCKS the absorption of Copper... That is a short-term approach that has significant long-term implications...

Cipro is activated with Fluoride...

Fluoride is a poison...

Fluoride ravages Mg status in the body...

Folks, MTHR NATURE'S natural "anti-biotic" is called CuZnSOD... it requires healthy levels of Copper and Ceruloplasmin...

It is easily checked with a blood test...

It is correctible with a nutritional program to restore the Liver's production of this critical protein that ensures the bioavailability of Copper...

It requires that you suspend your "D"evotion to certain very vogue, but equally as toxic, Hormone supplements that are ALL the rage right now...

MJ Hamp suggests: If you do not have access easily to an essential or macerated oil of Oregano...... here's what I would do:

Go into the kitchen and grab that jar of Oregano, open the jar and dump it into a cup and add a bit of hot water.... twice the amount as the herb. Let it sit about 30 minutes. Take a bit of the mash and put it on a band-aid and apply it to the soles of your feet.

It will not take long to taste it in your mouth.

For you gardeners.... fresh is best. Just go out to the garden and cut a good handful.

Anxiety

There is NO such thing as "general anxiety disorder..." GAD actually stands for "Glutamic Acid Dehydrogenase" I'm assuming that you know that. But in case you still believe this condition comes via "bugs from Mars," here's the metabolic TRUTH of its origin:

http://alcalc.oxfordjournals.org/.../37/6/513.full.pdf

This is an obscure, but INCREDIBLY accurate, assessment of the origin of these symptoms -- published in a HIGHLY respected and stuffy medical journal and clearly notes that ALL this mess stems from nutritional deficiencies as noted in Table 2 and it's also worth really studying the dynamics of these nutrients in Figure 2:

o   Maggie...

o   B1: Thiamine...

o   B2: Riboflavin...

o   B3: Niacin...

o   B6: Pyridoxine...

And what causes these nutrients to leave the scene or misbehave?...

"Stress!"...

And what's the antidote to "Stress!"?... Why yes, none other than our sponsor, Maggie:

http://www.ncbi.nlm.nih.gov/pmc/articles/PMC3198864/

Unfortunately, this ain't Rocket Science, although many, many, many practitioners -- the world over -- strive MIGHTILY to have us believe that it is...

And the OTHER side to this dynamic is to understand that this GAD Enzyme, is highly sensitive to Oxidative Stress:

http://onlinelibrary.wiley.com/.../j.1471-4159.2001.../pdf

So, what's this 3rd article ^^^^ saying?...

When you have sufficient bioavailable Copper, your body and your brain can produce optimal levels of anti-oxidant enzymes to NEUTRALIZE Oxidative Stress, not the least of which is CuZnSOD...

And how does Copper become "bioUNavailable?..."

Chronic "Stress!"....

Hmmmmmmmm...

Rising levels of ACTH and Cortisol KILL the production of Ceruloplasmin (Cp) the critical protein to ensure Copper's bioavailability...

Please take the time to familiarize yourself with the metabolic origin of these "GAD" symptoms -- ALL are borne of mineral deficiencies, especially Mg and Copper... It's time for Mo' people to know this TRUTH...

Our Ancestors had the luxury of going to the Mountains or the Sea Shore to imbibe in the relaxing settings (and eat mineral-rich foods...) of those popular vacation spots... That ambiance, coupled with the "OFF" button, does wonders...

A luxury that seems to be lost today....

I'm a bit battle weary from soooo many folks who have severe mineral deficiencies as profiled on HTMAs and subsequent blood testing. And the conventional course of Tx is Benzo's!...

OMg!!!...

Those that are seeking an alternative view to conventional dogma seem to find value in my nutritionally-oriented responses...

Folks who are "hyper-sensitive" are the unfortunate intersection of Mg deficiency AND Copper dysregulation...

It requires a dual approach to balance the minerals overall, and especially these two key agents (Mg and Cu) that keep us "Calm" when happy, and keep us on "Edge" when not...

Bugs, Critters and Guests (Pathogens)

Humans have co-existed with ticks for the last 6,000 or 6 million years (depending on your persuasion...) it's been in the last 50 years that our "immune systems" have been unable to marshal a response...

Hmmmm...

Given that minerals run the immune system, and that minerals have been disappearing at a voracious rate during that same time period.

It's time to arise from the "slumber" and see the world as it really is, not as the media is portraying it... We are, indeed, living "1984"... And while you may not like it, Black is white, and White is black... It's that stark!

Humans and ticks have co-existed on this Planet for a loooooooong time...

What's changed is our innate defence mechanism to KILL the bacteria and the parasite associated with these symptoms. Historically, that has been done by Superoxide Dismutase and Catalase...

Contemporary Humans are now Copper deficient and thus LOW on these Copper-dependent anti-oxidant enzymes...

There is waaaaaaay more to the story than your Mineral Denialist druggist is telling you or even knows...

With increasing frequency, I'm realizing that Copper dysregulation is lurking in the background with incredible precision...

And the MAJOR clue is to start Googling: "Your Favorite Chronic Disease" with "Oxidative Stress"...

And the code is that LACK of bioavailable Copper is at the CORE of Oxidative Stress... It plays a KEY role in:

- o SOD (Superoxide Dismutase)
- o CAT (Catalase)
- o GSHpx (Glutathione Peroxidase)

The failure to understand the essential role of Anti-Oxidant Enzymes in FIGHTING bugs, critters and guests has been one of our biggest short-comings...

Not anymore.

Clinical signs of LOW bioavailable Copper:

- o Lyme
- o Excess ammonia production
- o Excess glutamate
- o Kryptopyrroles

Time to re-think what's holding back your metabolism...
I've written extensively about this dynamic here on MAG and on the Copper Dysregulation and Rebalancing Facebook group...

It requires understanding the blood levels of

- o   Plasma Zinc...
- o   Serum Copper....
- o   Serum Ceruloplasmin....
- o   Iron- all 4 facets...
- o   Magnesium RBC…

It also requires that you understand that Copper is NOT a toxin, despite the fact that 98% of ALL articles re this mineral would indicate such...

What's KEY to this issue is that the Anti-Oxidant Defense system that routinely KILLS bugs, critters and unwelcomed guests -- when there is sufficient levels of bioavailable Copper... That is NOT the case with folks around the Globe...

Regrettably, this is a delicate and complicated subject that requires patience, persistence and tenacity to work through.

Not the "quick" answer you were expecting, but it's the $64 million question that we should ALL be asking our doctors...

Please know, there are two schools of thought about addressing Lyme disease:

- o   Nuke the bugs (attack the "guests")...
- o   Rebuild and strengthen the immune system (strengthen the "host")...

The latter requires a strong protocol based on minerals and immune support, which draws heavily on Maggie being at the top of her game...

I, for one, do not believe that the Good Lord invented "Biofilms" to mess with us... I may be widely out of touch with conventional practitioners for that statement and stance, but I'm a firm believer in allowing the body to restore its immune function, particularly since we have co-existed with tics for 6MM years, and the ONLY change in the last 50 years has been the capacity of our immune system to fight disease naturally...

The body is being constantly assaulted by "guests..."

This idea that there are "diseases" and "infections" is a lingering misconception that was crafted by Louis Pasteur 150+ years ago. That notion of the "Germ Theory of Medicine" should have died with him, but it is a pernicious "virus" that won't stop -- despite the fact that he was a total scientific fraud. (Check the NY Times for that article in 1995...)

In any event, the body's innate ability to NEUTRALIZE the Free Radicals is the essence of health... And it is DEPENDENT upon minerals...

Given that we LOSE Mg, Zinc, B-Vitamins and Copper to "Stress!", it might be worthwhile to re-read that article and assess the extent to which those conditions might apply when you were carrying your child in your womb, or whether exposure to noxious toxins like vaccines could have tipped the scales in her well-being...

Regrettably, it is SIMPLE mineral deficiencies that have been swept under the rug and replaced with fancy sounding "Latinese" Labels, and because we're human, that makes us gullible, and we believe all this silly nonsense re "disease" and "infections" -- not realizing that it's a function of our nutrient status, shaping our innate immune system...

Cancer

http://alignlife.com/articles/toxicity/millions-falsely-treated-for-cancer-says-national-cancer-institute-report

Hope everyone takes a moment to read this sobering and distressing article...

Please note the admission that those with cancer are "nutrient deficient..."

Can anyone guess what mineral is RAVAGED by Cancer Treatment, whether it be:

o   Chemotherapy..
o   Radiation Therapy...
o   Surgery...

ALL CAUSE Mg DEVASTATION...

Also, 90% of folks who die, don't die from Cancer, but from malnutrition induced by a severe lack of digestive enzymes, ALL of which are Mg dependent...

(All is NOT as it seems...)

People with cancer have elevated levels of UNbound Copper AND Anemic levels of Catalase (CAT)...

What's with that?...

o   CAT is the natural, innate enzyme that the body uses to KILL cancer cells... It's a well-proven mechanism as Marsha is pointing out...

o   CAT can ONLY be made when there are sufficient levels of Bound Copper...

o   What's a proven way to prevent Copper from binding to Cp (Ceruloplasmin)?... HIGH doses of Ascorbic Acid!

So HIGH AA "mimics" the H2O2 function of CAT and ensures that 30 other Copper enzymes are kept deficient for LACK of properly bound Copper...

AA, the perfect stealth agent for dis-ease and metabolic dys-function...

It boggles the mind, eh?!?...

Candida / UTI / Immunity

UTIs are CAUSED by Oxidative Stress!

http://www.ncbi.nlm.nih.gov/pmc/articles/PMC1533893/

SOD and CAT are BOTH dependent on bioavailable Copper for production and activation... Yes, CAT is billed as "Iron-dependent," but happy bio available Copper makes for happy bio available Iron.

I'd be checking your Cp status, along with Serum Copper and Iron, Copper RBC (a key measure of CuZnSOD) all of which may be low...

Also, I'd up your intake of wholefood Vit-C, and see what in your routine might be interfering with the production of Cp...

It would appear that D-Mannose works BECAUSE of Copper:

http://pubs.acs.org/doi/abs/10.1021/ja00706a020

Don't get me wrong, I'm heralding the use of D-Mannose (new arrow in my Quiver), but let's be sure to KEEP the spotlight on the MINERALS that run the body...

Also, Candida does NOT like ESOD (Erythrocytes) and LSOD (Leukocytes), BOTH of which are Copper-dependent:

http://jn.nutrition.org/content/120/12/1692.full.pdf

I know that it's a bit much to believe, but the LACK of bioavailable

Copper is ABSOLUTELY at the CORE of why our immune systems are so "anemic!" and incapable of neutralizing the Oxidative Stress being produced by the invaders...

However, please know that ALL manner of bugs, critters, yeast and PARASITES CAVE to the macrophage BURST of innate human killer cells with optimal levels of usable Copper that then ENSURE optimal levels of CuZnSOD to fire up our immune system...

Tragically, MOST health practitioners -- Allopathethic and Alternative -- trained with Bill Murray at "Caddyshack Medical School" and will resort to ALL SORTS of "attacks," when all that's needed is some focused understanding of how to control these infections by strengthening the HOST...

I'm modeling MY medical school after this SAGE and FOCUSED healer Down Under:

https://www.youtube.com/watch?v=RZy3ASozmk0

Here's my take on why SOOOOO many women, especially are struggling with immune issues:

o   You were raised on a LOW Fat diet... (Copper is BEST absorbed with Saturated Fat... Fat is BEST metabolized with Copper... Hmmmmm...)

o   You were raised on Antibiotics -- for the SLIGHTEST infection. (ABX BIND up Copper, KILL ALL bacteria and lead to Yeast overgrowth...)

o   Many were raised in homes that have Copper pipes

carrying acidic water that leaches Copper into our bodies (Yet another source of unbound, unusable Copper...)

o   Many have used Soy and Soy-based products (including being "bottle-fed" with Soy-based formula) completely overlooking the influx of yet MORE Copper that is NOT usable to the body due to a lack of Cp or inability to make sufficient Cp...

o   Many -- Lancet (2013) puts the current estimate at 48 million women -- use Birth Control Pills or Copper IUDs... (BOTH flood the body with excess, unbound Copper)

o   Many -- Almost ALL my clients! -- bought the BS that Hormone-D was their "salvation!" and are NOW dealing with sub-basement Potassium, virtually NO Vitamin-A and LOW Ceruloplasmin (Cp) function that is ESSENTIAL to fire up the bioavailability of Copper...

LOW Cp coupled with HIGH unbound Copper is a BAD combination... for countless metabolic pathways, not the least of which is our immune system...

Is it just me, or does anyone else see the OBVIOUS manipulation of the immune system to BIG Pharma's benefit?!?...

MTHR NATURE'S anti-dote to Candida is called "bioavailable Copper!" It is what enables the production of CuZnSOD, which is a CRITICAL enzyme that Red Blood Cells and White Blood Cells use to KEEP CANDIDA IN CHECK...

The vast array of info on the Internet and FB Groups creates the illusion that this or that is ALL that's needed to "fill that nutritional/functional gap..."

This is what I've learned since 2009:

o   Restoring Mg status is basically "self-serve..."
o   Addressing Copper dysregulation is akin to a "tune-up!"

I wouldn't DARE try that without a trained and competent "mechanic..."

You really need to know whether you are a "Fast" or "Slow" Oxidizer, which is BEST determined via an HTMA. No, I'm not trying to be an HTMA Pimp, although it appears that way. I am NOT aware of any other "definitive" way to determine this status. And targeted blood testing is then ADVISED to get into the weeds of how your body is working with its metals:

https://requestatest.com/mag-zinc-copper-panel-with-iron...

Once we've got ALL that, then we get down to the 20-point plan to restore Ceruloplasmin (Cp) production in your Liver which is where MOST of the problem REALLY is...

It would appear that most, if not all, gut dysbiosis is CAUSED by Copper dysregulation and Iron overload... The lack of bioavailable Copper leads to a lack of anti-oxidant enzymes, principally SOD and CAT, and this then leads to an increase in Iron-induced "Oxidative Stress!" which is usually involved in these conditions, certainly IBS, Crohn's, Colitis, etc.

Copper RBC is a surrogate for CuZnSOD... I can assure you your doctor has NEVER ordered that test before...

Cholesterol

I'll let you in on a little secret... What CAUSES "familial cholesterol" is familiar DEFICIENCY of Copper...

o   The mineral imbalance of your great-grandmother's Placenta created your Grandmother...

o   The mineral imbalance of your grandmother's Placenta created your Mom...

o   And, so on...

o   And what is supposed to happen in the Last Trimester of a pregnancy is that the Mom is supposed to infuse the foetus's Liver with 10X more Copper and Iron than they will carry as an adult...

It is NEXT TO IMPOSSIBLE to have sufficient bio-available Copper in an era when we live with:

o   Soil that LACKS Copper due to NPK fertilizers... (Nitrogen BLOCKS Copper uptake...)

o   Food that lacks this mineral due to the starved soil...

o   Prevalence of Anti-biotics (90% of ABX are used in Commercial farming...) which BIND UP Copper...

o Prevalence of ubiquitous High Fructose Corn Syrup (HFCS) that CAUSES LOW Copper and High Iron in the Liver... (High Iron SHUTS DOWN Copper metabolism...)

o Obsession with Hormone-D only supplements that CAUSE a decline in Liver Retinol, a critical precursor to MAKE Ceruloplasmin, KEY to making Copper usable...

o Prevalence of Glyphosate that is BOTH a mineral chelator (Mg and Copper) and an Antibiotic... Hmmmmmmm...

Other than these reasons ^^^^ there's no reason why we should be short on Copper in our tissues...

It "appears" genetic -- but, in fact, we are witnessing a generational DECLINE in Copper in our environment, despite the fact that we are being overwhelmed with forms of Copper that are UNUSABLE in the body...

Copper metabolism is indeed, a "Cu-nundrum!"

The metabolic issues of the Heart revolve around making energy... It is the ONLY muscle that works 24/7/365...

o It is HIGHLY sensitive to "Stress!"

o "Stress!" CAUSES Mineral Loss, especially Mg and Zinc.

o Energy is spelled Mg-ATP, and under "Stress!" the Mg DROPS OFF causing a DROP In precious energy in a muscle that thrives on it!

o   When "Stress!" Becomes chronic, Copper loses its protein, Ceruloplasmin, which is KEY to having usable Copper and Iron...

o   Copper is ESSENTIAL to MAKE ATP inside the Mitochondria...

o   When ATP cannot be made, free radicals get produced which cause a DROP in pH...

o   Low pH burns up Mo' Maggie!... which causes Mo "Stress!" and Mo' Loss of Minerals...

o   The elevation of Cholesterol is CAUSED by low levels of usable Copper (Klevay LM, 1982)...

o   "Stress!" CAUSES a DROP in Cp which makes Copper NOT usable...

o   Lack of bioavailable Copper CAUSES an increase in Lipid Peroxidation which we know as "Plaque!"...
     - because unmanaged Iron increases Lipid Peroxidation...
     - because bio-available Copper prevents the production of KEY Anti-Oxidant enzymes to PREVENT/STOP Lipid Peroxidation.

o   The BEST thing to do to PREVENT and RECOVER from a Heart Attack is to KNOW and BALANCE your minerals, especially, Mg and Copper...

o   The WORST thing you can do is ignore the minerals and take Rx Cardiac Meds... Why?!?

o   They CAUSE Mg loss -- across the board! (No, that is NOT a typo...)

Given the issues with High Cholesterol, it might be safe to conclude that you're dealing with low levels of bioavailable Copper and axcessed unmanaged Iron...

The recent back-to-back of Dental Surgery AND Eye Surgery has only intensified the "Stressors!" adding to your LOW Copper: (Cortisol STOPS Liver production of Ceruloplasmin (Cp)...

https://www.jstage.jst.go.jp/.../jser/68/1/68_1_9/_article

(At least the Abstract's in English...)

A new angle for you to pursue is to explore increased levels of Oxidative Stress and how THAT would be contributing to your vertigo...

The Anti-Oxidant Enzymes (SOD, CAT, and GSH) are heavily dependent on bioavailable Copper... As the free radicals build, these reduced oxygen species (ROS) *ding* DNA structures and metabolic enzymes in the inner ear that are likely contributing to your lack of balance dynamic...

EVERYTHING that's "booga-wooga" about Cholesterol is BIG Pharma induced "fear porn!"

100%!

Please read this carefully:

http://m.jn.nutrition.org/content/130/2/489S.full.pdf

Complex Reginaol Pain Syndrome (CRPS)

Let me come at this from a slightly different perspective...

I'm not familiar with this condition, but it is triggered with Oxidative Stress and resolved with anti-oxidant enzymes, as you likely know...

Here's the result of my brief research:

o   Here's the link connecting CRPS to Oxidative Stress: http://www.ncbi.nlm.nih.gov/m/pubmed/22798149/

o   So what we know is that Nrf2 plays a key role in Anti-oxidant Enzymes: http://ac.els-cdn.S2213231713000645-main

o   Ah, but it turns out that Nrf1 and Nrf2 have a relationship with Copper, which I suspected: http://www.ncbi.nlm.nih.gov/.../PMC39.../pdf/nihms560555 .pdf

o   Then we learn that low bioavailable Copper affects GSH http://www.ncbi.nlm.nih.gov/m/pubmed/8116544/

o   Life Extension has a good overview on Liver Detox and highlights many products that stimulate Nrf2: https://www.lef.org/.../metabolic-detoxification/page-02...

o   Finally, this overview of a naturopathic approach for NF (neurofibromatosis) seemed relevant, as well: .

My take on this is that your friend is NOT dealing with CRPS, but has a raging LACK of bioavailable Copper, and it's likely that your doctor(s) have NEVER thought to look there. Most don't, due to their scripted medical education...

Key to this dynamic is knowing the serum level of Ceruloplasmin, coupled with knowing you Zinc, Copper and Iron status, will shed important light on WHY the Antioxidant Enzymes (SOD, CAT, GSH) are NOT doing their job. More often than not, its from the mineral catalyst (Copper) being missing...

Minerals are akin to the keys that *start* our cars... And enzymes work the EXACT same way as the engine in our cars...

And very often what can block the critical functioning of this important mineral is the presence of Heavy Metals, most notably, Mercury... Be sure that she's not dealing with a toxic load there as Mercury has a special affinity for Copper-dependent enzymes...

Hope that helps and as you have further questions, please ask away!

Forget everything you "think" you might know about this condition...

Ground yourself in UNDERSTANDING three aspects of those articles:

1)   That Oxidative Stress CHANGES the performance of KEY Enzyme pathways...

2) That bioavailable Copper is the lynchpin in the body to run and activate these KEY Enzyme pathways...

3) That Copper becomes bioUNavailable under conditions of chronic "Stress!" which causes the Liver to slow/stop the production of the protein, Ceruloplasmin (Cp), which is essential to make Copper bioavailable...

Given that, read and ask away...

I've now identified 20+ factors (and COUNTING...) that are critical to the optimal production of Cp in the Liver...

Maggie, of course is just ONE of them...

Steps to Increase Ceruloplasmin (Cp):
o STOP Hormone-D ONLY Supplements (KILLS Liver Retinol needed for Cp)
o STOP Calcium Supplements! (Ca BLOCKS Mg & Iron absorption...)
o STOP Iron Supplements!.(Fe SHUTS DOWN Cu metabolism...)
o STOP Ascorbic Acid (It disrupts the Copper<>Cp bond)
o STOP HFCS & Synthetic Sugars (HFCS Lowers Liver Copper)
o STOP LOW Fat Diet (Fat is needed for proper Copper absorption)
o STOP Using Industrialized, "Heart Healthy" Oils!
o STOP Using products w/ Fluoride (toothpaste, bottled Water, etc.)
o STOP Taking "Mulit's" & "Pre-natals" (They have 1st four items ^^^^)

o START CLO (1 tsp Rosita's or 1 TBSP Nordic Naturals) for Retinol (Vit-A)
o START Mg supps to lower ACTH & Cortisol (Dose: 5mgs/lb body weight)
o START Wholefood Vit-C (500-800 mgs/day) - source of Copper
o START B8 (Biotin) -- Key for Cu/Fe regulation in Liver
o START B2 (Riboflavin) -- Key for Cu/Fe regulation in Liver
o START Boron -- 1-3 mgs/day (aids in Synthesis of Cp)
o START Taurine to support Copper metabolism in the Liver
o START Ancestral Diet (HIGH Fat & Protein/LOW Carb)
o START Iodine (PREQUISITE: Mg & Se RBC need to be optimal)

Dementia

Likely this is fueled by Aluminum Toxicity... Yes, good, clean saturated fats (especially, coconut oil, as noted above..) and good proteins, solid minerals, focus on Maggie and ATP Co-Factors (Carnitine, D-Ribose and CoQ-10) will be key...

If you haven't done a Mag RBC, this would be essential to assess how big a metabolic climb you have.

And Vegetable Oils are pure poison. Any oil "bottled" in clear plastic is rancid.

Period!

Mag oil IS NOT an oil. It is Mg Chloride which has an oily feeling to the touch, although it is a salt...

MgCl "oil" is dehydrated Seawater and "feels" slippery...

Toxic, "heart healthy," vegetable oils are the product of an 18-step process to convert "Seed Lipids" (a true Fat!) into a liquid that works wonders inside your body, especially after its been sitting in sunlight for a couple of months, which exellerates the oxidation (rusting) of the oils...

No two substances could be farther apart in their metabolic function, nor their biochemistry...

Health @ Mach-1: MgCl oil
Disease @ Mach-2: Veg. Oils!

Frederick A. Kummerow, PhD, a 100-yr old Lipid Biologist STILL actively researching and publishing, would agree that "industrialized oils" are NOT for the health of our heart...

Not even a schmidgin!!!....

Depression

This study is a penetrating look into the obvious... They have KNOWN since 1928 that Mg deficiency CAUSES Depression...

One of the many THOUSANDS of jobs in the body/mind is for Mg to sit NATURALLY in the NMDA Receptor... it is KEEPING you from excitation in those receptors.

When Mg is PUSHED OUT due to "Stressors!" -- Calcium takes its place and CAUSES pain... It's WELL documented in the literature...

Please read this to better understand the Mg Loss <> "Stress!" Connection:

http://www.ncbi.nlm.nih.gov/pmc/articles/PMC3198864/

The Mg loss is CAUSED by "Stress!", the perception of "Stress!", and SSRIs... (No, that is NOT a typo...)
The loss of Mg does NOT follow the stopping of these drugs... As for Benzo's -- ALL bets are OFF... They are among the MOST neuro-toxic and "D"estructive Rx Meds on the Planet.
They, and ANY Mineral Denilist that prescribes them, should be shuttled OFF this Planet -- permanently!...

http://evolutionarypsychiatry.blogspot.com.au/.../Magnesium

Benzo's RE-WIRE the Glutamine<>Glutamate<>GABA chemistry, in large part by disrupting Copper metabolism...

They ALSO affect Mg metabolism... I'm still trying to sort it out, but know that folks who are coming off Benzo's have to be careful with Mg, Cu, and B-Vitamins -- among other supplements.

That is NOT normal, NOR natural for the human brain to be "REACTIVE" to these foundational nutrients as supplements... I would advise you to reach out to Gidget Arrowood Day who understands this Benzo issue 100X better than me...

She is mineral-aware, most compassionate, and a damned fine musician!...

The natural response is to restore mineral status... I have learned thru painful trial and error that MTHR NATURE has been tweaked by these drugs... Regrettably.

Also, I would say that the MORE food-based the nutrients, the more the body/mind knows what to do with it... Synthetic supplements from a "B"ottle are NOT the answer, despite our familiarity and desire that they be... Remember, who owns 95+% these supplement companies?...

Not to depress you... but I've been working with folks on nutritional issues and mineral restoration for the last 7 years... Hands down, the most challenged and most compromised by the TOXIC, Allopathetic industry are those that have been hosed by Benzo's...

Those that predicate then are a pyrrha to society... Period.

Be patient and persistent... and you will overcome this imbalance.

I would also strongly encourage you to read this article by George Eby, PhD:

http://cureyourdepression.wordpress.com/.../magnesium.../

What you will learn is that ALL depression is CAUSED by an imbalance of Calcium and Magnesium...

Despite your belief that "hormones can cause depression..." please know that Adolf Butenandt, PhD, the German Physiologist who received the Nobel Prize in 1939 for discovering (Isolating) the first human hormones (Androgen, Estrogen and Progesterone) declared that ALL HORMONE IMBALANCE WAS CAUSED BY AN IMBALANCE IN Calcium and Magnesium...

Hmmmm... (Not and insignificant observation)

Fibromyalgia

Mg Malate, Mg Glycinate and Mg Cl are likely the best forms to restore Mg status to offset the condition of Fibromyalgia. Another useful product would be ATP Co-Factors made by Optimox in CA...

http://www.optimal.com

A Mg factoid...

Oxalates go into solution 567 X faster with Maggie than with Calcium. (And a million X faster than Mercury...) It's interesting that so often folks are told to take "Calcium Citrate" prior to/with meals... On the basis of the above, that seems questionable...

Please know that some of the BEST insights about Mg emerged in the golden era of 1950-1980 -- before BIG Pharma took control of medical research... and world-wide, some of the BEST research is coming out of labs in France, Italy, Japan, New Zealand, India, etc.

ANYWHERE but in the United States, with the notable exception of Burton and Bella Altura, PhDs (SUNY Downstate Medical Center) who have modestly published 1,000+ articles on Maggie and Mg deficiency in their illustrious careers...

HealthWatch news clip on local television reports a study that vitamin D is helpful for Fibromyalgia Syndrome (FMS).

Here is my response:

https://www.facebook.com/WLNSTV/posts/588452684567774

A couple of relevant comments...

Guy Abraham, MD, FACOG was a HUGE proponent of Mg to solve all manner of issues in his distinguished OB/Gyn practice and has numerous articles to prove that. Vit-D was never a part of his protocol. An important article to understand his perspective is:

http://www.mgwater.com/gacontro.shtml

It's worth considering that Hormone-D is the OLDEST hormone on this Planet... Hmmmmm...

Now I realize that I'm a total nudge on this issue, but the research is more and more supporting the FACT that hyper-supplementation of synthetic "D" is NOT warranted, nor healthy. And if you don't believe that, please take a spin through the FILES to find ample evidence to support that statement...

I'll let the master speak to this key issue...

http://www.westonaprice.org/cod.../cod-liver-oil-basics

Please enjoy both the article and the FCLO...

The confusion abounds because scientists, practitioners and writers do NOT identify the specific form/stage of Hormone-D that they are talking about...

o   Dehydrocholesterol: "Vit-D" is Cholesterol under the skin...

o   Prohormone-D is what gets created AFTER Dehydrocholesterol... mixes with Mg...

o   Cholecalciferol is what gets created AFTER Prohormone-D...mixes with Mg...

o   Calcidiol (Storage form of Hormone-D) is what gets created in Liver with Mg...

o   Caltriol (Active form of Hormone-D) is what gets created in our Kidney...

Depending on the writer, ALL OF THESE DIFFERENT FORMS is called "D3!"

No wonder we are all hopelessly confused...

Did you notice a certain mineral is in the thick of CREATING each of these forms of "D?"...

Please know, the physiological origin of INFLAMMATION is Mg deficiency (Weglicki and Phillips, Am Jrl Physiol, 1992).

What a coincidence...

A major factor in CFS/fibromyalgia is the inability to produce energy (spelled Mg-ATP) INSIDE the body and inside the cells...

Here's an important article that will explain how Magnesium plays a key role in that process:

http://www.mgwater.com/gafibro.shtml

That's the energy side of the equation...

As for the Allergy/Histamines issue, it's likely that you've got a condition called "Copper Dysregulation" which is a mineral conundrum of too little bio-available Copper and too much unbound Copper that disrupts Histamine function... And what causes Copper to be "unbound" from its target protein, Ceruloplasmin? Well, it's a lack of energy (Mg-ATP!) Imagine that...

Here's another important article since you're in the zone that will explain everything about Copper that your Doctor likely never told you...

http://www.westonaprice.org/mentalemo.../metals-and-the-mind

Please know, there are three topics that doctors will NEVER talk about: Magnesium status, Copper Dysregulation, and Adrenal Fatigue. And that troika accounts for the VAST majority of chronic disease that afflicts folks the world over...

Please feel free to keep asking those "newbie" questions! It's why we're here and it's how we ALL learn the truth...

o   The NMDA Receptors are designed to have Magnesium... When folks are swimming in Calcium -- because we have been ill advised to take Calcium until the cows come home, never telling us that it PREVENTS Mg uptake...

hmmmm -- that causes these pain receptors to "fire" wildly, which is adding to pain...

o   Furthermore, it appears that salicylates are aggravated by Mg deficiency and Zinc deficiency...

http://link.springer.com/article/10.1007/BF02795332

That's a new twist, but it plays into the likely imbalance of Calcium: Magnesium that is driving this issue...

http://www.mgwater.com/seelig_magnesium_deficiency_with...

Please know, the FASTEST way to deplete your Maggie is to drink a "Diet Coke!"

o   pH = 2.5 and must be buffered with Maggie and Potassium...

o   Synthetic sweeteners are a toxin that requires Mg to Detox

o   Phosphates EAT MAGNESIUM FOR LUNCH...

o   Artificial colors... more toxins, that need to be detoxed...

Those are the headlines...

The human species is NOW the Rat in the largest experiment to induce mineral deficiency and see how long they can keep taking toxic, but costly, Rx meds and keep the cash register ringing...

You think I jest?!?...

America spent $1.6 Trillion on Healthcare expenditures in 2004. The REST OF THE WORLD spent $1.2 Trillion...

(Please let that sink in...)
And drum roll please...........

Our health status is 37th of the top 40 Industrial Nations...

Major Hmmmm...

American "tax" dollars at work...

FDA rejected Aspartame for 16 years straight until Donald Rumsfeld was Secretary of Defense, demanded his buddy be the FDA Commissioner who tipped the vote in favor of its approval and the rest is history...

Just another dark chapter in that agency's stellar track record of Funding Death and Autism in America!

Fibromyalgia is the INTERSECTION of MO' Pain and No Energy...

o   MO' PAIN: NMDA Receptors are kept calm by Maggie in the saddle of these KEY receptors... when "Stressed Out!" Maggie takes flight and CALCIUM gets in the Saddle and CREATES Pain...

o   No Energy: The rate-limiting step in the production of ATP in our Mitochondria occurs at Complex IV, when Cytochrome c Oxidase gives up its electrons to Oxygen and CREATES ATP. That KEY enzyme is Copper-dependent (despite the fact that Iron is present)

Furthermore, the body does NOT recognize this key energy molecule unless it is "spelled" Mg-ATP inside the cells... Said another way, THERE IS NO ENERGY ACTIVATION UNLESS ATP IS COMPLEXED WITH MAGGIE...

Now, here's where it gets FASCINATING...
HORMONE-D:

o	puts a metabolic DEMAND on Maggie... it's a drain on this precious metabolic mineral...

o	It's JOB in the body is to ABSORB more Calcium and PLACE it in the blood -- at the expense of Maggie...

o	Hormone-D and Retinol (the TRUE form of Vitamin-A in the Human...) COMPETE for absorption... Said another way, if there is ONLY Hormone-D coming in, it will cause a LOSS of Vitamin-A...

o	Vitamin-A is a CRITICAL precursor to the production of Ceruloplasmin (Cp), an ESSENTIAL protein that makes Copper usable...

o	Increased intakes of Hormone-D ONLY will CAUSE Copper to be unusable...

Sooooo, we have Hormone-D:

o	Increasing the activator of Pain -- Calcium...
o	Decreasing the minimizer of Pain -- Magnesium...
o	Decreasing the neutralize of Mg - -Iron...
o	Decreasing the CREATOR of ATP -- Copper...
o	Decreasing the ACTIVATOR or ATP -- Magnesium...

There is NO way that Hormone-D is "good" for Fibromyalgia.

Fluoride and your water

The three MOST Toxic elements on the Planet, according to the EPA (with maximum allowable amounts...)

o Cyanide: 1 part/billion
o Fluoride: 4,000 parts/billion
o Lead: 1 part/billion

Oh goodie! They've lowered the maximum allowable by 50% -- BFD! (Big Friggin' Deal)

Poison is STILL Poison -- at ANY concentration!

FLUORIDE IS POISON. PERIOD...

Another important factor is knowing the pH of your originating water... It does make a difference and acidic water will leech Copper -- just as it does in MOST homes with Copper piping, but that's because most water is NOT pH 7.0 as it should be...

We use Berkey filtered tap water, with Prills, in our home and office...

(http://www.health-and-wisdom.com/)

Then Jazzed up with either Andersons Mineral Drops (84 minerals) or Aussie Mineral Drops (92 minerals)...

Don't leave home without it!...

Please know, the bodies "go to" mechanism to CONTROL pH is the status of Magnesium and Potassium inside the cell...

Also, one of the most important enzymes in the human body to ensure proper pH is Alkaline Phosphatase...

You'll be happy to know that this enzyme MUST have Mg to work properly...

This is especially important for bones, heart, liver, kidney, brain, and a few other parts of the body that depend on this enzyme...

A large part of WHY we're so acidic has to do with the inability of this enzyme to work properly. It is the key reason for Osteoporosis, as Osteoblasts (bone matrix builders) MUST work in an alkaline environment.

Where you might be at a disadvantage is that you are relying on "current, and contemporary" textbooks and research. Trust me, the Mg message and importance has been artfully censored from most of the documents you're perusing...

The older the research, the more revealing and accurate it is. The cutoff date is ~1984 when BIG Pharma took over funding the medical and pharmaceuticals research in the U.S.

I wish you the best in the launch of your new integrated venture. I would only ask that if you do nothing else, please get a Mag RBC on each and ALL of your clients. That one blood marker is the gateway to virtually every other blood marker... and I'd be happy someday to explain that to you and your colleagues...

I realize that minerals, and especially Maggie, are a bit boring and basic. But unfortunately, the human body runs on them. It's biologic. Focus on the mineral foundation and you'll be amazed at how the sophisticated metabolism of the human species corrects its problems -- on its own...

That we are even having this dialogue is DEFINITIVE PROOF that we are Circus Bears in the midst of "1984!" -- Where Black is white, and White is black:

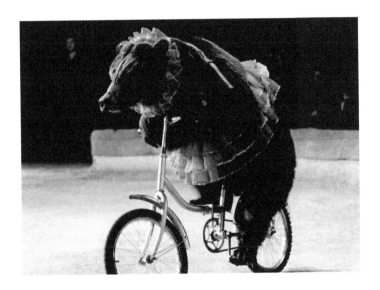

o   We are being TAUGHT to fear Magnesium...
o   We are being TAUGHT to feed Fluoride -- wherever possible!...

The truth of the matter:

o   Magnesium:
http://www.ncbi.nlm.nih.gov/.../pdf/1471-2105-13-S14-S10.pdf

o   Fluoride:
http://www.nofluoride.com/.../nobel%2520prize%2520winners

For heaven's sake, FLUORIDE is POISON. Period! Buy three copies of this book:

http://www.amazon.com/The-Devils-Poison.../dp/1425144845

One for YOU to read... One for you to give to this Bozo, DDS, (whom you should FIRE!) and, one for your NEXT DDS to read BEFORE allowing them to touch your teeth...

Wake up folks! It's POST "1984!" Black is white and White is black...

Hashimoto's

Hashi's = Autoimmune = XS Oxidative Stress = too little antioxidant enzymes = TOO LITTLE BIOAVAILABLE COPPER...

You do NOT have a "medical disease..." You DO have "metabolic dysfunction" CAUSED by "Stress!"-induced "mineral deficiencies..."

That's a VERY different dynamic and lack of usable Copper affects energy pathways, immune function and a wide swath of symptoms that get many, many, many "labels" from the Mineral Denialists that have NO KNOWLEDGE of the role and function of minerals in the human body...

That FACT alone should make us ALL quiver at the thought of asking them to "heal" us!...

Best way to raise your D3 levels:

o   Take Mo' Maggie...
o   Eat Mo' Fat!...
o   Get Mo' Sunshine...

We were NOT designed to increase this hormone by eating irradiated sheep skin oil...

In the REAL world...

o   Hashi's and MTHFR are expressions of Copper and Iron dysregulation...

o   Low Calcidiol (25(OH)-storage-D) is proof positive of Mg deficiency:

http://gotmag.org/vitamin-d-deficiency-mg-deficiency-period/

Trust me, Mg deficiency and Copper dysregulation are your issue, Hormone-D is PURE "D"istraction, in my humble opinion...

The tests that are warranted:

http://requestatest.com/mag-zinc-copper-panel-with-iron...

http://requestatest.com/mag-vitamin-d-panel--testing (Have them pull out the duplicate Mag RBC)

http://gotmag.org/work-with-us/

I would investigate Copper dysregulation (Oxidative Stress!) and/or Mercury Toxicity. Also, if there are unresolved "Stressors!" in your environment, they are most effective at depleting Maggie...

This is the "Stress!" Pathway likely involved:

"Stress!" = Mg Loss = High Cortisol = Low Ceruloplasmin (Cp) = High unbound Copper = Low SOD (anti-oxidant) = High Oxidative Stress = Low Maggie

Hypothyroidism and Your Moons

"Hypothyroidism" is a mineral imbalance: Excess Calcium and too little Potassium. How does that occur?

When we get "Stressed Out!", we lose our Maggie...

Oh, I'm aware of the need for Iodine, Selenium and Iron for proper Thyroid function, and that the T4>>T3 conversion gets impaired... But far too few practitioners know that:

o   Magnesium and Copper are key to putting on and taking off Iodine,

o   That the Selenium-activated enzyme is DEPENDENT on Mg-ATP, and that selenium absorption is DEPENDANT on bio-available Copper......

o   That virtually every aspect of Iron metabolism is Copper/Cp dependent...

o   That the T4>>T3 conversion gets blocked by too much Cortisol in the system -- CAUSED by too little Maggie, as well as Oxidative Stress in the Livers...

o   That the T4>>T3 conversion ALSO gets blocked by too much unbound Copper -- CAUSED by too little Maggie...

Anyone seeing a pattern here?!?...

For those that don't know, one of the principal roles of Synthroid is to LOWER Calcium in the body... Hmmm. Why that's the VERY job of Magnesium -- it is Nature's Calcium Channel Blocker... That has been proven time, and time again, and denied consistantly by BIG Pharma and their Minion Deities...

And yes, according to multiple (5+) Oriental medical sources, "Moons" are associated with:

o   Chi, our overall energy status

o   Oxygenation of the blood

o   B-12 status

It was our clients who began re-gaining their Mg status and noted that their Moons were growing back -- much to theirs and our surprise... So, we backed into realizing that "Moons" are aligned with Magnesium status because there are three things that must have Mo' Maggie:

o   Chi, overall energy status... (No Maggie, No Mg-ATP, THE unit of energy in the body...)

o   Oxygenation of blood (enzymes to put on and take off Oxygen are fueled by Mg-ATP...)

o   B-12 transport INTO and OUT OF the cell is dependent on Mg-ATP...

Hmmmm...

Again, anyone seeing a pattern here?!?...

Mg-ATP is THE unit of energy to run ALL 100 Trillion cells of our body.

You can NOT make energy without Magnesium.
You can NOT recycle energy without Magnesium, and you can NOT activate energy without Magnesium.

Any time you see "ATP" in an article or scientific literature, it is missing its FULL expression "code" for Mg-ATP. ...

And the most amazing thing is that your doctor is TOTALLY unaware of this physiological FACT.
And how do I know this?!?

Because virtually every Rx med that is used today is classified as "Magnesuric" -- which means CAUSING Mg LOSS IN THE URINE... And MAG FB Group is heavily populated by many, many folks dealing with that very physiological phenomenon as evidenced by the majority of Mag RBCs that are BELOW 5.0mg/dL (bottom of the Functional Range)...

Please know, there are 149 Kinase Enzymes that virtually run the cell. They are ALL dependent on Mg and Mg-ATP. There is one, CaMKII (calcium/calmodulin/kinese II) that requires Calcium. Its job: bring the cell to death (Carlo, 2014)...

Cells do NOT act independent of their mineral masters... It's that basic. Cellular metabolism is built on a mineral foundation. Period. We are 72% H2O and 28% Minerals... and EVERYTHING our bodies run on depends on those two classes of elements. Without energy (spelled Mg-ATP) there's a whole lot of metabolic dysfunction that occurs...

So, again, focus on the mineral foundation and try not to get seduced into thinking that there are more important, more sophisticated, or more complicated things than minerals that provide the stimulus, electrical charge, pH, etc. to enable us to have optimal health...

By the way, "Moons" on pinkies are a sign of Heart Disease, according to numerous Chinese Medical sources...

Here's a listing of the "Stressors!" from your note above:

o   Parents divorced, family "Stress!"

o   Involved in a highly competitive and dangerous sport...

o   Baaaaaad accident...

o   2 Surgeries (exposed to Fluoride activated Anesthesia...)

o   Anti-Biotics (they are Magnesuric, and affects Copper and Iron Status!)

o   Pain meds are Magnesuric!

o   Being "flat on your back," and NOT on a horse!

o   Involved in a marital relationship, however supportive, is stimulous for "Stress!"

o   Restricted food diet

And all of the above (and what we don't know...) creates mineral imbalances that then CAUSE:

o   Leaky Gut
o   Set the stage for Lyme (due to weakened Anti-Oxidant Enzyme Defense)...
o   Hypothyroidism (High Calcium/Low Potassium)...
o   Gluten sensitivity

Besides physical trauma, another accepted cause of "Beau's Ridges" is metabolic dysfunction:

http://www.medicinenet.com/beaus_lines/symptoms.htm

From what I understand about Metformin, it's real impact is to create an increase in Lactic Acid, which is very hard on the cell. Lactate Dehydrogenase, a key enzyme to keep Lactic Acid in check, is stimulated by excess unmanaged Iron...Please note, an increase of Lactic Acid revolves on Mg status...

Lyme Disease

The body is being constantly assaulted by "guests..."

This idea that there are "diseases" and "infections" is a lingering misconception that was crafted by Louis Pasteur 150+ years ago. That notion of the "Germ Theory of Medicine" should have died with him, but it is a pernicious "virus" that won't stop -- despite the fact that he was a total scientific fraud. (Check the NY Times for that article, in 1995...)

In any event, the body's innate ability to NEUTRALIZE the Free Radicals is the essence of health... And that is DEPENDENT upon minerals...

Given that we LOSE Mg, Zinc, B-Vitamins and Copper to "Stress!", it might be worthwhile to re-read that article and assess the extent to which those conditions might apply when you were carrying your child in your womb, or whether exposure to noxious toxins like vaccines could have tipped the scales in her well-being...

The critters of Lyme HATE the innate Anti-Oxidant Defense system of our Immune System... But it ONLY works when there is sufficient levels of Bioavailable Copper...

Either your doctor doesn't know that or doesn't want you to know that... (Which is the GREATER sin?!?...)

Regrettably, it is SIMPLE mineral deficiencies that have been swept under the rug and replaced with fancy sounding Latinese

Labels, and because we're human, that makes us gullible, and we believe all this silly nonsense re "disease" and "infections" -- not realizing that it's a function of our nutrient status...

Please also refer to the Bug, Critter and Guest Chapter.

MTHFR

The fact that a condition is "popular" and "in vogue" is RARELY an indication of its alignment with metabolic truth...

MTHFR is VERY popular and VERY sexy... it's complicated, it's confusing, it's CONTEMPORARY...

I put my stock and trust in MTHR NATURE, not a contrived "pseudo-science" that appears "real" because it's SOOOO detailed, but fails to fully speak to and account for the mineral dysregulation that CAUSES the Transcription error...

Sometimes, it's REALLY important to look BEHIND the Green Curtain, a la "The Wizard of OZ" and see what's REALLY going on...

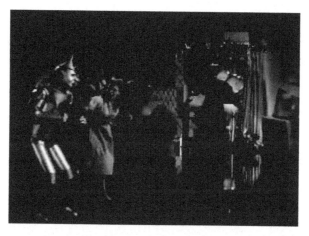

The Methionine Synthase enzyme is Copper dependent -- that's the Head Enzyme of the MTHFR dynamic...

Wait, you mean ALL this MTHFR dynamic is CAUSED by epigenetic "Stress!" from MISSING MINERALS?!?...

Be still my heart...

My concern is that the world of MTHFR is Looooooong on WHAT, and very short on WHY... It's most distressing to a guy seeking to enlighten the masses about how MTHR NATURE REALLY works...

Yes, you do have epi-genetic "Stress!" CAUSING it... Yes, you do need Mo' minerals to support that process...

No, I do NOT think synthetic B-Vitamins, methylated in a test tube, is the answer...

Bioavailable Copper via Ceruloplasmin is SUPPOSED to do that naturally...

And TOTALLY ignores the KNOWN effect that Mercury has to BLOCK Copper metabolism -- you knew that, right?...

And yes, I'm just a curious blogger, with apparently better critical thinking skills than most, and have pulled back the "Curtain of Deception" on COUNTLESS metabolic processes, and nutritional regimens... Why?...

Because I think its HIGH time folks KNOW that minerals RUN the human metabolism -- not Rx meds!

No, I don't have a bunch of degrees, and certificates to validate what I have to say, I rely on the 2500+ scientific articles that I have read and synthesized since 2009...

Yes, I do have clients in 30 countries who seem to think I know what I'm talking about... Apparently, sanity and success spreads like wildfire...

To delve deeper I would INSIST on TWO ground rules:

1)   Discussion grounded in ENZYMES and the minerals that activate them...

2)   Discussion of WHY the minerals got tweaked...

I am no longer interested in the WHAT of MTHFR...

It's time we get to WHY and HOW...

In my humble opinion...

Beware MTHFR... You'll become as crazy as a Mad Hatter trying to sort that out...

Focus on the mineral foundation to understand how the human metabolism REALLY works...

MTHFR is ALL about WHAT...

It's not until you get to the mineral deficiencies that CAUSE the transcription errors and lowered availability off activating enzymes that you get to WHY...

In the REAL world...

o   Hashi's and MTHFR are expressions of Oxidive "Stress!" Born of Copper dysregulation...

o   Low Calcidiol is proof positive of Mg deficiency:

http://gotmag.org/vitamin-d-deficiency-mg-deficiency-period/

OMg!

ENZYMES ARE EVERYTHING!

And what makes enzymes work?

MINERALS!

Just like your car, they do NOT work unless the mineral KEY is present...

And in the case of SAMe, it is nothing without Maggie and B6 -- this "amazing" video FAILED to paint that foundational truth.

Furthermore, it was silent on the FACT that Methyltransferase (MT) enzymes are Copper dependent - - at least the 10 that i have studies carefully (COMY, HNMT, PEMT, etc.) I'm making the leap that MTHR NATURE would use that catalyst in ALL MT enzymes...

Hmmmmmmm...

So for anyone seeking to transcend their bondage of ME/CFS, those would be two excellent minerals to start with: Mg and Cu!

The purpose of MAG is to spread TRUTH, NOT further the deception and disinformation of BIG Pharma.

Again, our message and our purpose at MAG is MINERALS, 1st and FOREMOST!

I know this idea that "Lithium is key to B12" has been popularized within the MTHFR community, but Lithium is a true micro-nutrient, very little is needed. Mg-ATP, which is ESSENTIAL to activate the enzyme to get B12 INSIDE the cell, is a rapidly disappearing concept in the homo americanus... Especially with those who are dealing with Adrenal Fatigue...

Again, I go after the most obvious causes...

http://www.ebi.ac.uk/thornton-srv/databases/cgi-bin/enzymes/GetPage.pl?ec_number=3.6.3.33

Multiple Chemical Sensitivity (MCS)

The "label" MCS is masking the fact that your polyphenol oxidase enzyme is lacking bioavailable Copper...

This is a classic Histamine Intolerance response, and the degradation of Histamines REQUIRES Mg, Cu and B6. If there's too much "unbound" Copper, it will KILL Mg and B6 due to its pro-oxidant qualities...

Mg is important, and Copper being properly bound to Ceruloplasmin (Cp) is absolutely CRITICAL in this dynamic. Please know, MCS is NOT a "medical disease..." that is pure Allopathic witchcraft!

Heavy metals, especially Mercury, have a unique affinity for Copper and Copper dependent enzymes... Mercury has "estrogenic qualities" and Copper is the mineral that activates the enzyme to MAKE Estrogen...

Copper dysregulation is at the core. It is mind-numbing, but Copper dysregulation is at the core of MOST chronic conditions... And "Stress-induced!" LOSS of Maggie starts that Copper dysregulation dynamic...

I'll do my best to address this issue with you...
Over reaction to your environment Polyphenol Oxidase (Copper dependent) enzyme is likely over-reacting to the environment:

http://link.springer.com/article/10.1007%2Fs00726-005-0298-2

Failure to do so, sent you into what is likely a Histamine Intolerance reaction:

http://ajcn.nutrition.org/content/85/5/1185.full.pdf+html

Be sure to study Fig 1, carefully...

An HTMA plus these blood-based mineral markers that will reveal what's going on:

https://requestatest.com/mag-zinc-copper-panel-with-iron...

As for, "can my GP do this?..."

There are two seesaws:

o   If your GP orders these tests, you save $$$, but will lose Mg (as they will question you or get it wrong, esp. the Mag RBC -- 98% of the time they do...)

o   If you use Request A Test, you lose $$$, but your GP saves their Mg as they won't show up on a Quality Review Panel ordering "weird blood tests..." nor have to deal with the embarrassment of NOT knowing how to properly interpret the tests!

Those are your choices...

In my humble opinion, your Mg retention is WAAAAAY more important to you, so I'd belly up to the bar and pay for it out-of-pocket!...

But that's me...

There is TREMENDOUS PRESSURE for "D"octors to "D"o what they are TOLD TO "D"O... They have precious little latitude to do what's in the patients' best interests, despite hoe grating and offensive that may appear...

Please re-read that ^^^^ again to fully understand what's going on... Again, we are living "Post-1984!"... The world of medicine is NOT as it seems...

Now if memory serves me correctly, Liver detoxification, Phase I is ruled by Glutatione, GSH, which is dependent upon Sulfur, Selenium and there are two steps involving Mg-ATP to make that precious detox molecule. What is not entirely understood is that GSH seems to work best in the presence of bioavailable Copper, likely due to its role in firing up GSH-Peroxidase and/or GSH-Reductase...

Given the penchant that metabolic bully of the body, Mercury, has for Mg, Zinc and Copper, it would make perfect sense that Phase I would be tweaked -- assuming my memory serves me correctly...

I focus on lowering the environmental/metabolic "Stressors!" that lead to epi-genetic dynamics that cause the transcription errors. I'm not a Luddite re MTHFR, and recognize the importance of this testing and its impact on the selection of supplements. However, I do not buy that we're "broken." Please, also address the "Stressors!" and proceed accordingly...

You might find this article that I wrote helpful:

http://gotmag.org/mg-deficiency-affects-mthfr-really/

I would investigate Copper dysregulation (Oxidative Stress!) and/or Mercury Toxicity. Also, if there are unresolved "Stressors!" in your environment, they are most effective at depleting Maggie...

"Stress!" = Mg Loss = High Cortisol = Low Ceruloplasmin (Cp) = High unbound Copper = Low SOD (anti-oxidant) = High Oxidative Stress = Low Maggie

Likely you've been under notable "Stress!" which has depleted your mineral status, which then goes onto decrease the effectiveness and responsiveness of your Adrenal Glands, that sit atop the Kidneys and are your body's 1st line of defense to a toxic/stressful world.

Keep in mind, that during periods of "Stress!" we lose copious amounts of Mg, Zinc and B-vitamins, and then under chronic "Stress!" Copper leaves the body, as well...

Reaction to chemicals/perfumes is a classic sign on Histamine Intolerance, which aligns with the above, as these chemicals (Histamines) are designed to save you from the environment, but when we are LOW in Mg, Cu and Vit-B6, we are no longer able to breakdown the Histamines and we over-react to our environment.

Here's an outstanding article on this issue, please keep in mind that they are TOTALLY silent on the mineral dynamics behind this problem:

http://ajcn.nutrition.org/content/85/5/1185.full.pdf+html

You might pay particular attention to Fig 1 that might align with other issues that you are dealing with.

Bottom-line: you need to assess and re-balance your minerals.

Pediatric Heart

Becoming a Pediatric Heart Surgeon is laudable, but you might want to also read Stephen T. Sinatra, MD, FACC: "Metabolic Cardiology."

That book comes the closest to explaining the origin of so-called "heart disease" that is consuming folks globally. At the end of the day, the Heart, the most metabolically active tissue in our bodies, MUST HAVE ENERGY, which is spelled Mg-ATP... And the myopic fear of fat, coupled with a methodical elimination of minerals (especially Magnesium and Copper), has led to an energy crisis the global population has never witnessed...

This might be a great place to ground your clinical endeavors...

The most powerful step you can take as a Pediatric Surgeon is to FIRST measure the Mag RBC of the child (and their parents...).

The Reference Range for Healthy Homo Sapiens is 5.0-7.0 mg/dL (USDA Whitepaper on Magnesium, 1962). Any value BELOW 6.0 is a definitive sign of Mg deficiency. No, I don't know why this has never been a part of your clinical training...

Particularly when you consider the fact that >50 cardiac enzymes are activated by Mg and/or Mg-ATP...

Hmmmmm...

Pregnancy

The creation of new life is a roiling sea of minerals, vitamins, proteins, hormones, etc... As Mildred S. Seelig, MD, MPH, the world's authority on Magnesium, stated eloquently:

"Pregnancy is a Magnesium deficient state..."

The cause of so much crisis in the Delivery Room that is related to Pre-eclampsia (HBP) and Eclampsia (Seizures) is related to surges of Cortisol, signaling "Stress!" And when Cortisol is HIGH, it is a given that Magnesium will be LOW!...

And that is why Mg SO4 is the agent of choice in those situations.

But heaven forbid pregnant women assess their Mg status with a Mag RBC AT THE OUTSET OF THE PREGNANCY... and then monitor it throughout the trimesters...

For those that put a great deal of "stock" in their Pre-Natal vitamins, you might check with the manufacturer to assess the ppm (parts per million) of Fluoride that it contains...

Not to mention the water systems are "toxic" when flouride is above 4ppm. There are some of these supplements that are as high as 230ppm. Excess Calcium and Iron, the elevated Hormone-D and the fact that B-Vitamins are all synthetic.

I wish I were kidding...

Please read these:

http://www.ncbi.nlm.nih.gov/m/pubmed/20005782/?i=3

And here's the Motherload of WHY it's ESSENTIAL:

http://www.mgwater.com/.../Magnesium.../Chapter2.shtml

Please get a Mag RBC ($49 @ Request A Test) and start taking Mg Oil baths EVERY night...

Also, you might take a spin thru here:

http://gotmag.org/how-to-restore-magnesium/

Please not the fine print of MAG FB Group state:

o   If it's a girl, her middle name is Maggie...

o   If it's a boy, his middle name is Max... (Betcha thought I was gonna say "Morley!"...)

Mom's lose 10% of their mineral mass making the bambino...

During the last trimester, Moms infuse 10X More Copper and Iron into the Foetus' Liver than they'll carry as an adult...

Pre-eclampsia is a clinical sign of Mg deficiency, most likely from excess, unmanaged Iron. Also, please keep in mind that apples don't fall far from trees -- your "bundle of joy" is likely low on Maggie, as well...

Pre Menstrual Syndrome

o   Inflammation is CAUSED by Mg deficiency (Weglicki and Phillips, 1992)

o   Guy Abraham, MD, FACOG identified 4 types of PMS -- ALL were corrected with Mg and Vit-B6

o   Oxidative Stress is likely at play which is a sign of Copper deficiency, and as this article clearly states, herbs ROCK:

http://www.biomedcentral.com/content/pdf/1472-6882-14-11.pdf

Turmeric is rich in Maggie and I'm guessing Copper given its healing properties...

So, I'm all ears and eyes to learn what you feel is a better option. And thank you for bringing this issue to light for the benefit of the group...

o   Heavy menstruation is a lack of Retinol (animal-based Vit-A)

o   Anemia is a clinical sign of Copper deficiency...

I'm willing to bet you take Hormone-D, which is killing your Liver's Vit-A, which is preventing the Liver's production of Ceruloplasmin (Cp), which is CAUSING the lack of bioavailable Copper, which is the reason for your anemia.

And if you're taking Iron supplements for that, please know you are shutting down your Copper metabolism...

Post Traumatic Stress Disorder (PTSD)

MAG-pie Alert!... R.E.S.P.E.C.T

Dr. Liz and I had the pleasure of attending a Zydeco Dance Festival, to celebrate Memorial Day!... It's been a while since we've had THAT much fun, and danced THAT much!...

But, what was most memorable was watching a 95 yr old veteran, who served on submarines during WW II, doing a Cajun two-step -- with grace, ease, and delight in his eyes...

We don't often get a chance to experience that kind of vigor, and all too often what is associated with Veterans today is their struggle of re-entry due to PTSD. It's really quite sad, as this issue is TOTALLY a dynamic of "Stress-induced!" Magnesium deficiency. And this is well documented by one of my favorite nutritionists, Byron J. Richards, CCN.

Noted below is his summation of this metabolic issue of Mg loss with PTSD, and below that is the original research by William B. Weglicki, MD, one of my all-time Mg researcher heroes who has distinguished himself with his 2 decades of truth re Magnesium and Mg deficiency!

o   Connecting PTSD to Mg deficiency:

http://www.wellnessresources.com/.../magnesium_is_essential_.../

o   Original research by William B. Weglicki, MD referred to ^^^^

http://www.jle.com/.../--mrh-287106-
the role of magnesium def...

So, let's ALL take a moment to thank these men and women, throughout our lives, who have served their country, and the many who have offered their lives in return for our freedom. And for those returning Vets who are now challenged by the "Stress!" of their military experience, let us offer them hope and the truth via this powerful message re Maggie -- the mineral of metabolic recovery and balance...

Pyroles

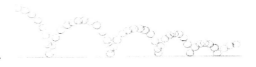

Follow the bouncing ball...

o   The conventional Tx for H.pylori is anti-biotics...

o   Anti-biotics BIND Copper...

o   Copper dysregulation is often at the center of many
     chronic conditions... Between your overall 'Stress!",
     illness "Stress!", and the added "Stress!" of "fast sugar,"
     your body and mineral balances sound in need of a tune
     up!...

Here's my letter to a client challenging the conventional treatment
of Pyroles...

I'll look forward to the "blow back!" Pursuant to our discussion,
I'm attaching a link that explains the METABOLIC ORIGIN of
Pyroluria:

https://pyroluriatesting.com/about-us/

What is very relevant is their assertion on Page 2 that:

"Any source of oxidative stress can elevate urinary pyrrole levels.
Many persons have elevated pyrroles resulting from factors such
as physical accidents, illnesses, infections, emotional trauma and
toxic metals."

This is a MAJOR TILT!...

It's very important to understand that chronic "Stress!" will result in elevated levels of ACTH (key "Stress!" hormone, and that will result in STOPPING the production of Ceruloplasmin (Cp) in the Liver, which then undermines the bioavailability of Copper.

Given that Copper plays a pivotal role in giving the Anti-Oxidant Defense pathway its potency (via the key antioxidant enzymes SOD, and Catalase), the WORST thing you could do would be to "DROWN" the body in Zinc, as that will only PREVENT Copper absorption and undermine the body's ability to mobilize an appropriate and consistent anti-oxidant response.

http://www.ncbi.nlm.nih.gov/pubmed/16112185

(Copper is THE key mineral for optimal anti-oxidative potency...)

The added insult is their assertion that Pyroluria is a:

"Chemical imbalance involving an abnormality in hemoglobin synthesis." What they FAIL to indicate is HOW IMPORTANT bioavailable Copper is to the optimal synthesis of hemoglobin.

http://www.ncbi.nlm.nih.gov/pubmed/16406711

(Ferrochelatase, the rate-limiting enzyme to MAKE Hemoglobin will NOT work without Copper...) In my world, the focus should be to CORRECT the Copper dysregulation, and NOT TREAT the symptoms that result from "Stress!"... In a word, this approach to "Pyrroluria" is just more "Affagato!

If you seek to distinguish yourself in the field of nutrition, here's my advice: Assume that the BULK of what they're cramming in your head is utter BS! Study minerals and the enzymes they empower and you'll rock the world...

Let's come at this with some data:

http://nutritiondata.self.com/facts/sweets/10638/2

Yes, there is a bolus of Maggie, but look at the %RDA for Copper, Manganese and Iron... YOWSER!

Those are three metals that are routinely tweaked in many, many people....

It's also important to recognize that most people with "high" Copper are often LOW, in reality, dealing with bioavailable Copper. And the fact that Phenyalanine Oxidase is a Copper dependent enzyme has fascinating implications.

I would caution you to think through the production of Heme and study the role of Copper in activating Ferrochelatase...

You might also study how defective Heme synthesis can lead to Kryptopyrroles, which THEN go onto to deplete Zinc and B6. It's also worth noting that elevated levels of bio-unavailable Copper have the same effect on Zn and B6.

Hmmmmm...

Once again, our boys in white lab coats have it Affagato (backwards!)

All that said, my $$$$'s on Copper being "craved!" And what's the SOURCE of craving?

Dopamine deficiency!

And how do you make DOPA? Take Tyrosine, add DBM enzyme AND Copper et voila -- Dopamine!

Again, I believe Copper's the target. And as my main mentor, Rick Malter PhD, has taught me, "Copper is the mineral of obsession..."

Salt And Your BP

Does regular salt increase blood pressure?

Most likely, due more to the Chloride ion than the Sodium ion...

In fact, denying the human body of Sodium leads to an increase of Aldosterone, the OTHER "Stress!" hormone that no one knows about, that CAUSES Loss of Zinc and Magnesium => which helps accelerate HBP... Clever, eh?...

It's a package deal... all of the Electrolyte minerals play a key role in BP.

This is a quote from Larry M. Resnick, MD's paper in PNAS in 1984:

"We believe our observations remain quite significant and suggest intracellular magnesium as a biochemical regulator of the physiology and pathophysiology of blood pressure control in man."

Enlightened physicians who can see beyond their Rx pads regard Dr. Resnick's article as a seminal piece of research about BP regulation.

Know that there is NO $$$$ in a cure...

Here's the article should you wish to read the full report...

http://www.pnas.org/content/81/20/6511.full.pdf

Dare ya to share it with your Internist!...

I totally get it, but while there is soooooo much to "unlearn," there really is only ONE thing to learn:

"Magnesium RULES... Calcium ain't so cool..."

Once you master that, you've pretty much mastered:

o   Inflammation Pathway... (Mg prevents...)

o   Insulin Resistance... (Mg activates Tyrosine Kinase)

o   Hormonal Balance... (Dr. Butenandt said Ca/Mg ratio was key)

o   Blood Sugar regulation... (Pancreas depends on this same ratio...)

o   Energy Pathways... (Mg brings ATP to life!)

o   Detox Pathways... (Mg-ATP is key to Glutathione Pathway)

o   Mineral Balances... (Mg is the Conductor of the Cellular Orchestra of minerals!)

o   And, about 2,000 other functions we don't have space to discuss...

Pretty cool, eh?!?...

(Don't worry, I didn't believe it was THAT easy at 1st, either...)

Just remember, the more Mg deficient the individual, the more acidic their pH and consequently, the slower the Mg uptake... One of the Mg "Catch-22" is the MORE you need it, the MORE challenging the uptake recovery...That's not how i would have designed it, but that is the reality of recovery...

I'm just sharing what I've read and experienced with clients. No, I can't change the rules!...

For those who REALLY want to understand the relationship between Salt, Edema, the Electrolytes and Metabolism...

http://raypeat.com/articles/articles/salt.shtml

Ray Peat is a very insightful and highly controversial nutritionist that has consistantly challenged "conventional" thinking...

What changes have occurred in your MBR (magnesium Burn Rate)?... This is the holiday season when "Stress!" elevates in the most surprising of ways...

Remember, even excitement and joy can be "Stressful!"

Seizures

At the risk of sounding like another "one trick pony..."

o   Lack of Bioavailable Copper will cause a decrease in antioxidant enzymes...

o   As the ROS (free radicals) build, they will oxidize the GAD enzyme that is VITAL to convert Glutamate >> GABA...

o   As the Glutamates build, they will burn out the Magnesium -- due to their neurotoxic effect -- and THAT is likely what causes the Seizure...

As for the Porphyria, please delve into how Heme is synthesized... Ferrochelatase enzyme is Copper dependent...

And when it's NOT present, bad things happen...

My fervent wish is that folks DROP the Labels of Medical Convention and learn to pull back the curtain to REVEAL the mineral dynamics CAUSING the metabolic dysfunction that Mineral Denialists LOVE to call medical disease...

It's TIME to shift your focus to the REAL DEAL... Get out of the world of BIG Pharma...

Does that make sense to ANYONE else?!?...

Hope springs eternal...

Any Veternarian knows that a cow with Grass Tetany (known as "grass staggers" since the 1860's, mind you...) must get Mo' Maggie! And when they do, their "seizures" STOP.

Thyroid

Three of the greatest propaganda plants in society:

o   You've got a Thyroid problem, never mentioning that ALL
       Thyroid issues START in the Adrenals...

o   You need Mo' Calcium, especially Calcium on
       Steroids, aka Hormone-"D", never mentioning that excess
       Calcium SLOWS the Thyroid, BLOCKS Mg absorption
       and BLOCK Iron absorption...

o   You need Mo' Iron (because your Ferritin is low...), and
       never telling you that Iron Supplements SHUT DOWN
       Copper metabolism...

o   When Copper is bio-UN-available it PREVENTS
       Adrenal recovery...

Pretty slick, eh?...

It's ALL programming, and NOT based on science, despite the
presents of white lab coats, stethoscopes and test tubes...

True listening requires a willingness to change...

Most people are TOO STUCK to change course, or are
UNWILLING to adopt new habits and beliefs...

Can't save them all... we save the ones that are willing to listen...
This is a MUCH more compelling and definitive study done re the
impact of Copper deficiency on Thyroid function:

http://naldc.nal.usda.gov/naldc/download.xhtml?id=44230...

An HTMA Class led by Rick Malter, PhD, he introduced a new factoid: I knew that the Thyroid is RULED by the ratio of Calcium:Potassium. Rick noted that as that ratio gets more and more out of balance, it affects the functioning of the Thymus gland (Hmmmm... Center for Immune response...). Extreme Ca/K >> Hashimoto's... Intriguing thought. I plan to follow up with him today to discuss these concept further...

With all due respect to the thousands of practitioners who make quite a living "treating" "Thyroid Disease" (not "curing," mind you...), you've got to move BEYOND the conventional box that guides these treatments...

Each of the Endocrine Glands is RULED by a mineral ratio. Thyroid is Ca/K. And as the folks at STTM acknowledge, you CANNOT heal the Thyroid until the Adrenals are working properly...

Adrenals are RULED by the ratio of Na/Mg... Hmmmmm...

And MOST of the Thyroid dysfunction is occurring in the Liver where T4 is supposed to be converted to T3... What BLOCKS this? Usually, excess Cortisol and/or, excess unbound Copper.

And what keeps Cortisol in check and the Copper properly bound to Cp?!? Magnesium!... What a coincidence...

Please know, I am grossly oversimplifying it. I've assembled ~12 different reason why Thyroid function gets tweaked. No less than 8 involve LACK OF MAGNESIUM.

Who knew...

Reflux

http://acne.about.com/od/acnetreatments/a/spironolactone.htm

That is a WONDERFUL article on Potassium that sheds important light on "Reflux!"

Here are some added thoughts:

o The Na/K ATPase pump in EVERY cell is run by Mg-ATP. Folks under "Stress!" lose Maggie, the pump STOPS working, Na rushes in, AND Potassium rushes out...

o Folks under "Stress!" ALSO lose Zn and B-vitamins... They are ESSENTIAL to make HCl...

o When "Stress!" becomes chronic, the excess Cortisol kills Ceruloplasmin production, Copper goes rogue and unbound Copper KILLS Mg, Zn and B vitamins...

Hmmmmm...

o Most folks don't know this, but excess, unopposed Hormone-D supplementation CAUSES Renal Potassium Wasting... HTMAs reveal this time, and time, and time again!

o B12 supplements CAUSE loss of Potassium...

o ALL Rx PPIs CAUSE LOSS OF Mg and Zn! Prilosec carries a Black Box warning that it CAUSES Mg deficiency. For the FDA to REQUIRE that is HUGE—it must be really bad to warrant THAT!

What's a PROVEN anti-dote to Reflux?...

Apple Cider Vinegar!

It's a RICH source of Potassium!

Your Heart

Please take the time to read this article carefully:

http://jn.nutrition.org/content/130/2/489S.full

There is a great deal of opinion about how to address Heart Disease.

In my humble opinion, most of it is based either on a complete misunderstanding of Cholesterol, or a protocol by a very gifted scientist who apparently lacked an understanding of the TRUE molecular structure of wholefood Vit-C...

The LAST thing you need in your body is high doses of Ascorbic Acid, but I lack the degrees and Nobels to compete with Linus Pauling, PhD.

o   What your heart needs is bioavailable Copper...

o   What makes Copper bioavailable is Ceruloplasmin (Cp)...

o   What DEPLETES Cp is Ascorbic Acid:

http://jn.nutrition.org/content/117/12/2109.long

ALL is NOT as it seems...

Please take these 3 steps:

1) Please read this article slooooooowly...

http://gotmag.org/what-is-heart-disease-really/

2) Please take a moment to then read and act on this material:

http://gotmag.org/how-to-restore-magnesium/

3) Please then ask your doc these 4 key questions:

A) How many proteins MUST have Mg to work in the human body? (A: 3,751 proteins -- the next is Zinc @300...)

B) How many enzymes MUST have Mg and/or Mg-ATP to work properly? (A: 2,200+ enzymes...)

C) How many Kinase enzymes -- that run ALL of our trillions of cells -- MUST have Mg-ATP to work? (A: 149 out of 150 Kinase Enzymes...)

D) How many CARDIAC enzymes MUST have Mg and/or Mg-ATP for the Heart to work properly? (50+ enzymes... by the way, there are four Mg-dependant enzymes, just to regulate Cholesterol... More Hmmmm...)

And after your doctor gets a bit flustered NOT KNOWING ANY OF THIS, you might ask him WHY IS THAT?!?...

That's the very question that burns in my cranium daily... How does the ENTIRE field of Allopathic Medicine, and especially

Cardiology, NOT KNOW THESE BASIC FACTS OF HUMAN PHYSIOLOGY?!?...

It's almost like it was DESIGNED ignorance...

Please know, the Achilles Heel of Allopathic Medicine is their total lack of awareness, acceptance or appreciation of Magnesium metabolism:

o   How to measure it properly...

o   How to interpret Mag RBC scores properly...

o   How to assess symptoms of Mg deficiency... (MOST are!)

o   How to stop Mg's constant depletion in their patients' bodies (due to the constant use of Magnesuric Rx meds -- MOST cause this!...)

o   How to recommend steps to increase Mg status in the body...

o   And on, and on, and on, and on...

It's quite sad, really.

As Pierre Delbet, MD, noted French physician once said: "Magnesium is a food, NOT a drug..." And the overwhelming majority of MDs have NO clue what that means...

Known Reference Ranges for the Magneium RBC:

1962: 5.0-7.0mg/dL
2014: 4.0-6.4mg/dL (Kaiser, Quest, etc.)
That is a 20% DROP in an acceptable value in 50 years.

However, when your temperature rises just 4% (98.6 >> 102.)
You feel REALLY BAD, right?...

Think about <u>THAT 20% DROP</u> in intercellular Magnesium might
just be fueling the meteoric RISE in how bad everyone is
feeling?!?...

Yeah, me too!...
We're entering a new phase where we need to take total control
and rely on practitioners as a RESOURCE and NOT a priest...

I'll let Patrick Chambers, MD (retired Cardiologist) speak to the
issue of Mg and AFIB:

http://www.afibbers.org/resources/PCmagnesium.pdf

I have read over 1,000 articles on Mg and Mg deficiency and
have a special interest in Mg and the ...

The BIGGER the lie... the MORE we believe it.

It's a sad commentary of our times...

The MOST important test you can complete right now is a Mag
RBC... The MOST important book you can read right now is
either "Metabolic Cardiology" by Stephen T. Sinatra, MD, FACC
or The Calcium Lie II, by Robert Thompson, MD, FACOG.

Your heart is weakened by the fact that your Mg is TOO LOW,

and your Electrolytes are imbalanced in your heart -- and that's the source of your overall lack of energy (Mg-ATP).

The entire "your heart is blocked..." paradigm is a skewed distortion of reality. Heart Disease has been this nations #1 cause of death for over 100 years... (Please let that sink in for a moment...)

The rate of Heart Disease is escalating, despite the fact that 40% of medical expense goes to treat this condition, and despite the fact that $tatin $ales are bigger than most nation's operational budgets. And what have 100+ years of Cardiologists "over-looked?..."

The fact that the Heart is THE MOST METABOLICALLY DEMANDING TISSUE IN YOUR BODY. Translation: it requires the MOST ENERGY (Mg-ATP). And it's a fact that the highest concentration of Mg in the human body is in the Left Ventricle of our Hearts...

So, please, get that test, read up on the Energy Starvation theory of Heart Disease, and keep on Magging!...

The Pacemaker Cells of the Heart (yes, there really are such buggers...) are regulated by a Mg-dependent enzyme, MKK-4. It really responds to Maggie, and not synthetic, Magnesuric Rx meds... you might share that with your doctor...

http://www.ncbi.nlm.nih.gov/pubmed/2755217

By the way, scientists begrudgingly say (last sentence): "the Mg ion MAY have an antiarrhythmic effect..."
OMg! The ignorance and arrogance that rules our doctor's

training!!!...

The heart muscle responds very well to:

o ˙ Mg Taurate

o Mg Malate (Jigsaw Health)

o Mg Glycinate (Pure Encapsulations, Drs. Best)

Please know, for Mg to have the optimal impact, it needs Vit-B6, especially, to get INSIDE the cell. The Jigsaw brand has that built into its formulation...

In addition to those oral brands, you would be advised to drink Mg water, and use transdermal Mg Cl oil, either directly on the skin, or in foot baths (1/2 Oz.) or full baths (1 Oz.)

What also needs to be factored into these types of delicate dynamics, is a broader context of what the status of the "other" minerals are...

Mg can work wonders, but does not act alone, as we all know... A good tissue mineral analysis would be a key factor in this process...

EF (Ejection Fractions) of the Left Ventricle are ALL about measuring the ATP/ADP turnover in this part of the heart muscle. That Critical function is Mg-dependant.

Apparently, doctors were asleep (or mesmerized) when the instructors informed them that when Maggie is low (Mg RBC <5.0mg/dL) the ATP/ADP turnover slooooooooooows down and the EF gets smaller, and smaller, and smaller. C'mon folks this ain't "rocket science..." Nor is it a disease. It is PHYSIOLOGICAL IGNORANCE, in my humble opinion.

And any doctor that doesn't know that does not deserve to practice medicine, in my humble opinion. Stephen T. Sinatra, MD explains this VERY, VERY, VERY well in his book.

Another of the great Mg "Rock Stars" is Gerald W. Deas, MD. He happens to be the 1st African American to receive the MD degree in the State of New York...

http://www.downstate.edu/.../funds/deas_professorship.html

His great-grandmother was a slave in the South and taught him how they kept high blood pressure under control on the Plantation: 1 tsp of Epsom Salt (MgSO4) in a glass of grapefruit juice...

Good for what ails you!

It worked flawlessly then... It works flawlessly now...

The condition of "cardiomyopathy" tells you that your heart muscle cells (cardiomyocytes) are NOT getting sufficient Mg-ATP to satisfy their energy needs -- which are voracious! The heart muscle cells are the MOST metabolically active cells in the body...

Please Read this as a refesher:
http://gotmag.org/what-is-heart-disease-really/

PROCESS OF DISCOVERY

What a HTMA Can Tell You...

HTMA and Urine are both valid ways to assess mineral status. I've no experience with the latter and don't know whether the mineral ratios metrics are the same...

When working with minerals, absolute AND relative levels with other key minerals are KEY...

As you might expect, there are differences in mineral presence in hair vs blood vs urine. It is very rare to see mineral studies using urine. (And In my humble opinion, the ONLY reason why organized medicine despises HTMA is that it reveals TOO MUCH in the body's metabolic dynamics!)

http://biolab.co.uk/

Remember, it's NOT the lab report, but it's the interpretation that is key!

Difference between mag rbc and mg HTMA

A key point is, how stable is the Mg RBC test? You can't fully determine a person's "stress" response from just the Mg RBC, without the broad based mineral dynamics that are profiled in the HTMA

Some random thoughts...

o   Heavy metal poisoning puts an enormous burden on your Detox Pathways, which are energized by Mg-ATP. You cannot make Glutathione without Mg, and nothing happens until the pathway gets energized...

o   CFS/Fibromyalgia is multi-factorial, but the lack of Mg-
      ATP causes muscle fibers to get "grumpy,"(p*ssed off!)
      and the lack of Mg in the NMDA Pain Receptors (which
      gets replaced with Calcium...) causes them to fire
      "Pain," non- stop...

o   Hippocampus is the center for memory, and is highly
      dependent on Mg for memory (yeah, who knew?...) and
      is highly sensitive to Aluminum and Copper Toxicity,
      again, these poisons need to be Detoxed! -- using up
      more Mg-ATP...

o   Not holding adjustments is a sign of notable Adrenal
      Fatigue. For some reason, weak Adrenals cause
      ligaments and tendons to go lax... My partner, Dr. Liz (a
      NUCCA/network chiropractor), taught me that...

o   If your Mg is down, which is almost always is with
      CFS/Fibro, then your Electrolytes are not properly
      balanced and only add to the metabolic dysfunction
      taking place in your body...

OK, with those thoughts as a backdrop, beyond the HTMA,
here's what I'd be seeking:

o   RBC testing of Mg, Na, and K

o   "Ionized" Calcium test

o   ATP/ADP Turnover Ratio (Mg deficiency will cause this
      to tank!)

o   Serum Copper

o   Serum Ceruloplasmin (transport protein for Copper)

o   Plasma Zinc

o   1,25(OH)2 D3 (Active form, aka Calcitriol)

o   Free T4 vs Free T3

o   Estrogen vs Progesterone...

That combination would provide a wide spectrum of information. Truth be known, that set of blood markers is a bit redundant to the HTMA, but as a society we are "trained" to believe that blood is best...

Hope that helps and when your results are in, I'd be happy to shed additional light on the levels and what they might mean... Blood Results combined with HTMA will give you are great overview of health.

What A HTMA Can Tell You....

By Genelle Young

When I began my journey of mineral balancing, I felt the need to know the why and how behind the diagnosis. I had tried many other avenues before going down this path, and for the first time, the evidence was right there in front of me. The more I read the more I wanted to know. With the need to read it over and over again, for it to register I put this together....

It may not be 100% correct but from my research, is was what I would refer to to see the progress my family was having. It opened my eyes to a whole new exciting world. For the first time in my 37 years the proof was in the pudding.

Morley will tell you aim of the game is to be kissing that red line.

Hair Tissue Mineral Analysis has been openly available for about the past 40 years or so. It is widely used in biological monitoring, of animal species throughout the world and is being used more and more, for human metabolic assessment as well. When understood properly, it offers great potential to improve human and animal health at the deepest levels. It can also be used preventively, and for prediction of illness.

A HTMA will supply you with reliable data on more than 35 nutrient and toxic Minerals, and over 25 important Mineral ratios. With standard blood and urine tests, valuable health information is often not revealed. Nutrient Mineral imbalances or toxic Mineral excesses that may be affecting your health, will be discovered.

Minerals are the basic 'spark plugs' of life.

Minerals are essential for growth, healing, vitality and well being. Structural support in bones and teeth, need Minerals, they also are responsible for maintaining the body's PH and water balance, nerve activity, muscle contractions, energy production and enzyme reactions.

Modern farming techniques, fertilizers and depleted soils reduce the Mineral content of foods, stripping your bodies of essential Minerals as does, environmental pollutants, chemical food additives and stressful lifestyles. All having a detrimental effect on our Mineral balance and nutritional state.

Cardiovascular disease, high cholesterol, high blood pressure, migraines, learning difficulties and hyperactivity in children, are just a few of many health conditions that are aggravated by Mineral imbalances and toxic metal excesses.

Consequently, we need to test and monitor our nutritional status more than ever.

Balancing Minerals is a journey, best traveled with an intuitive translator. A HTMA is not a form of testing we would suggest to self diagnose, or interpret. Please read the following content to give you a better understanding of the process, not to determine your status personally.

I like to focus on the first four Minerals on the grid, Ca,Mg, Na, K , as things fall into place when they are in balance. The ratios help to better understand the weakness we need to support to bring everything together.

This is not a short journey and may take a year or more to balance, but results may be seen within 3 months. Remember it took years to reach your current status.

Ratios are more important than just levels. Ratios give us the bigger picture and are indicative of disease trends. Ratios are often predictive of future metabolic dysfunction. Ratios are a great tool for charting progress as whole picture, not isolating one ratio. There are five ratios we focus on:

Calcium/Magnesium (Ca/Mg) Ratio (Blood Sugar - Cardiovascular Health)

This is often referred to as the blood-sugar ratio and is an indicator of insulin status. Calcium is needed for the pancreas to release insulin. Magnesium inhibits secretion of insulin, so it is necessary to keep calcium and Magnesium in harmony.

Ideal ratio is 7.00, however 3.4 - 9.9 is good.

Below, 3.3 is indicating you are heading to Hypoglycemia, it would indicate Magnesium loss, with possible blood sugar issues, and perhaps a hidden Na/K inversion. With 2.5 - 3.3 meaning diabetic symptoms. Any lower than 2.5 would suggest, onset of symptoms such as mental and emotional disturbances.

Above, 110 again indicates you are heading to Hypoglycemia with, tendency to insulin resistance, relative Magnesium Deficiency and possible overeating carbs. 13-18 showing diabetic symptoms, lifestyle changes needed. Any higher than 18 would suggest, onset of symptoms such as mental and emotional disturbances. High Calcium will lower cell permeability, creating a "Calcium Shell"

Magnesium or Calcium loss will raise levels temporarily, many factors can make this happen, such as Cortisone therapy lower calcium levels and will also impact Sodium and Potassium levels by raising them. Calcium can become displaced by Lead and Cadmium toxicity. I don't like to focus on the area of toxicity and prefer to balance and let the body do its job, naturally.

Sodium/Potassium (Na/K) Ratio *(Overall Vitality)*

This is a crucial ratio and often referred to as the life/death ratio, because of its importance.

The electrical potential of the cell is regulated by Sodium and Potassium, and is related to the Sodium pump mechanism, both regulating Potassium and Sodium within our body.

The ratio is an indicator of the intimate relations of the Kidneys, Liver and the Adrenal Glands functions. An imbalance of this ratio is closely associated with the Heart, Kidneys, Liver and Immune Deficiency Diseases.

This ratio gives us an indication of the Adrenal Gland function, and the balance of Cortisone and Aldosterone.

2.4 is the ideal ratio, 2.9 - 3.9 is good.

4.0 - 12 is moderate, with above 12 being extreme. High ratio would indicate, alarm reaction, acute stress, inflammation, and anger.

2.0 - 2.3 is moderately low, with 1.0 - 1.9 being serve. Below 1.00 would suggest delusional, out of touch, decreased awareness of signs and symptoms, feeling like "you are beating your head against a wall".

Na is a rough indicator of Mineralocorticoid effect (Aldosterone), pro inflammatory) K is a rough indication, of glucocorticoid effect (Cortisol), anti-inflammatory)

Na ideal is 24 - 75 alarm - 75 resist - 10 exhaust
K ideal is 10 - 5 alarm - 30 resist - 30 exhaust
ratio ideal 2.4 - 15 alarm - 2.5 resist - 0.33 exhaust

Na/K is showing signs of going into resistance stage of stress, hence the Sodium up and Potassium has come down, means it is gearing up to turn to resistance stage then exhaustion stage.

Sometimes on retesting this ratio can show worse than before, as other Minerals work so closely in relation to these two. Change in Copper status, will change this ratio as will Increase in Magnesium.

Remember Potassium in needed for your bodies to process sugar, so until you are healed, avoid sugars.

Calcium/Potassium (Ca/K) Ratio *(Thyroid)*

The Thyroid ratio because Calcium and Potassium regulate the Thyroid. Often blood tests will indicate normal ranges, whereas the HTMA will foresee the issue. Often there will be symptoms of hypothyroidism, whereas the hair test will indicate hyperactivity thyroid ratio. This is where the whole picture needs to be taken into account.

4.2 is the ideal range, 3.0 - 8.00 is a good range, with 8.1-50 being moderately Hypo, and above 50 indicating extreme Hypo.

1.0 - 2.9 would indicate moderate Hyper, and below 1.00 extreme Hyper.

Low Ca (<30) would suggest hypersensitivity, hyperkinetic, anxiety, nervousness, muscle cramps, increased permeability,unprotected psychologically, tendency to Ca deficiency.

Low K (<4) would suggest body exhaustion, but mind keeps pushing, sense of "running on fumes" and Cu toxicity regardless of Cu level and if Ca is above 50.

Thyroid proceeds Adrenals. You will not balance Thyroid until Adrenals are supported.

Sodium/Magnesium (Na/Mg) *(Adrenal)*

This ratio is referred to as the Adrenal ratio, because our Sodium levels are directly associated with the function of our Adrenals. Aldosterone, a Mineral corticoid Adrenal hormone, which regulates retention of Sodium in the body. Corticoid is any of a group of more than 40 organic compounds belonging to the steroid family and present in the cortex of the Adrenal Glands. Higher levels of Sodium would indicate, higher levels of Aldosterone.

The Adrenal ratio also measures energy output, as the Adrenals are the major Gland of the rate of metabolism.

As with the Thyroid, often blood tests will not detect an issue with the Adrenal Gland, whereas the HTMA will show the imbalance.

4.00 is the ideal ratio, with 3 - 6 being good. 6.1 - 20 would suggest moderate elevation, with tendency towards inflammation. 20+ is severe elevation, resulting in inflammation and Adrenal imbalance. Asthma, allergies, Kidney and Liver issues can be related to high ratio, that being said, high is preferred to low.

1 - 2.9 would indicate mild Adrenal fatigue, with possible digestive issues, Kidney and Liver dysfunction, allergies, arthritis, Adrenal exhaustion, deficiency of hydrochloric acid. Below 1 can indicate a tendency towards heart attacks, cancer, as well as the above symptoms. It is the state of extreme Adrenal Fatigue/ suppression.

However in saying that there have been people with a ratio below one, that were functioning well.

Sodium levels can be elevated by excess levels of several Minerals including Mercury, Iron, Copper, Cadmium, nickel. These levels will be taken into consideration when reading your HTMA.

Zinc/Copper (Zn/Cu) (Female Hormones)

This ratio is an effective measure of zinc and Copper readings. Elevated levels are often associated with skin problems such as, acne, psoriasis, slow healing, and eczemas. Also, emotions instability, "spaciness", PMS. Reproductive problems, menstrual issues, depression and fatigue, schizophrenia.

8.00 is the ideal ratio, with 6.5 - 10.00 being a good range. 10.1 15 is moderately high, with 15+ being extremely high. High ratios can be deceiving because of hidden Cu. With hidden Cu, the symptoms of low Zn/Cu will be present.

3.0 - 6.4 is moderately low, with below 3 being extremely low. Fast Oxidizers usually have a true low Cu and Zn. Slow Oxidizers with a low Cu usually have low bio-available Copper and excess, unbound Copper which is quiet toxic to the body.

Calcium/Phosphorus (Ca/P) (ANS State - Protein Usage)

This ratio will indicate your body's ability to break down and use Proteins.

Phosphorus levels indicates Protein usage, protein reserves and tissue breakdown. When P is low or high the following questions need to be asked, is the client eating enough Protein, from good sources, and is digestion of proteins the issue, perhaps needing HCL??

Low P is worse the high, with impaired protein synthesis being worse with low Zinc.

Ideal range is 2.63, with 2.3 - 2.8 being in the good range. 2.9 - 8.00 is moderately high with 8 and above being extremely high, Anabolic processes.

1.5 - 2.3 is moderately low, and below 1.5 being extremely, Catabolic processes.

CURRENT IDEAL HAIR MINERAL VALUES
(hair must not be washed at the laboratory for accurate readings)

MacroMinerals:

Calcium = 40 mg%
Magnesium = 6 mg
Sodium = 25 mg%
Potassium = 10 mg%
Phosphorus = 16-17 mg
Sulfur = 4500 mg%

NOTES: Sulfur usually is a little higher in fast oxidizers, up to about 5000 mg%.

Trace Minerals:

Zinc = 15 mg%,
Iron = 2 mg%,
Copper = 2.5 mg%,

 = 0.03-0.04 mg%,
Chromium = 0.06 mg%,
Selenium = 0.12 mg%,
Cobalt = 0.002 mg%,
Lithium = 0.002,
Molybdenum = 0.002,
Boron = 0.05-0.08 mg%,
Rubidium = 0.06,
Germanium = 0.003,
Iodine = 0.1 mg%,
Vanadium = 0.004 mg%,
Zirconium = 0.005 mg%
Ideal Levels Of The Toxic Minerals:

Most important toxic metals:

Lead = 0.06-0.09 mg%,
Mercury = 0.03-0.04 mg%,
Cadmium = 0.005-0.007 mg%,
Arsenic = 0.005-0.008,
Aluminum = 0.65-1.0 mg%,
Nickel = 0.02-0.04 mg%

Other toxic metals (that are much less well researched):

Uranium = 0.002-0.004 mg%,
Strontium = .008-0.01 mg%,
Antimony = 0.005-0.01 mg%,
Barium = 0.03-0.05 mg%,
Beryllium = 0.001-0.002 mg%,
Bismuth = 0.05-0.1 mg%,
Silver = 0.08-0.1 mg%,
Tin = 0.02-0.04 mg%,
Titanium = 0.05-0.07 mg%,
Platinum = 0.008-0.01 mg%,
Thallium = 0.004-0.006 mg%,
Thorium = 0.004-0.006 mg%.

Raising Minerals by lowering other Minerals

To raise Mineral:	Lower:
Calcium	Potassium
Magnesium	Sodium
Sodium	Magnesium / Zinc
Potassium	Calcium / Copper
Zinc	Potassium (if Na/K is low)
	Sodium (if Na/K is high)
Chromium	Iron / Copper / Manganese
Manganese	Iron / Copper / Calcium

Iron	Manganese / Zinc
Copper	Manganese / Zinc

The added wickedness to Copper is that ONLY "Fast" Oxidizers (20% of the population) can take Copper supplements, and the ONLY way to assess your Oxidizer pattern is through an HTMA. The notable distinction is that the Fast Oxidizer has an ability to metabolize Copper "directly", while Slow oxidizers has an equal need for bio-available Copper, but it needs to be provided "indirectly" via Wholefood Vitamin C Complex, NOT Ascorbic Acid, NOR Copper supplements, as they will only "slow" the "Slow" Oxidizer even more.

The definition of a **Fast Oxidizer** is someone with a Calcium/Potassium ratio less that 4:1 and Sodium/Magnesium ratio higher than 4.17:1. A Fast Oxidizer releases energy too fast. A Fast Oxidizer has a tendency to burn through Slow minerals like (Ca and Mg), and retain Fast minerals like (Na and K)

The definition of a **Slow Oxidizer** is someone with Calcium/Potassium ratio greater than 4:1 and Sodium/Magnesium ratio less than 4.17:1. A Slow Oxidizer releases energy too slowly. A Slow Oxidizer has a tendency to burn through Fast Minerals (Na and K), and retain Slow minerals like (Ca and Mg).

Rarely there is a **Mixed Oxidizer** that will have a Calcium/Potassium ratio greater than 4:1 and Sodium/Magnesium ratio greater then 4.17:1 or Calcium/Potassium ratio less than 4:1 and Sodium/Magnesium ratio less than 4.17:1. A mixed oxidizer has an erratic metabolism, meaning sometimes too fast, and sometimes too slow.

The **Balanced Oxidizer** is where we want to be, when the main four, Calcium, Magnesium, Sodium and Potassium are in perfect harmony. Your body is provided with perfect constant useable energy. This is bliss, happy, content, open and uncomplicated. The Balanced Oxidizer possess an inner calm and balance.

Oxidizers Patterns: Fast vs Slow

Unfortunately, Copper is NOT a straight forward shot... No, it is NOT advised to take Copper supplements unless you are a Fast Oxidizer... and the only way to know that is to complete an HTMA and learn how you relate to the Electrolytes: Calcium, Magnesium, Sodium, & Potassium...

80% of folks are Slow Oxidizers and cannot tolerate Copper straight up... 20% are Fast Oxidizers and can do so... The best & safest way to restore Copper status is wholefood Vit-C Complex -- NOT Ascorbic Acid...

Believe it or not, Fast's oxidize the Slow minerals: Calcium & Mg... and hold onto the Fast minerals: Sodium & Potassium...

And Slows do just the OPPOSITE...

No, I do NOT know why some do it this way and some the other... It is the $64 million question in the world of minerals...

The added wickedness to Copper is that ONLY "Fast" Oxidizers (20% of the population) can take Copper supplements... And the ONLY way to assess your Oxidizer pattern is through an HTMA...

I am not sold on the parameters of the "Slow vs Fast" diet as it is based on a SUBJECTIVE questionnaire, and NOT purely objective science as you might have thought...

Let's Do An HTMA with Morley Robbins

o   Hair Tissue Mineral Analysis

http://gotmag.org/work-with-us/

o   Mg RBC (optimal is 6.0-7.0)

http://requestatest.com/magnesium-rbc-testing

o   Signs of Magnesium Deficiencies

http://gotmag.org/magnesium-deficiency-101/

o   How to Restore Mg:

http://gotmag.org/how-to-restore- magnesium/

Upon ordering you will receive an intake form and email from Morley ,and then via snail mail the HTMA kit, which will contain the necessary scale to weigh your hair sample. Please keep these scales as that will expedite future HTMA's. On the envelope it will say Shampoo and this is asking for the brand, as certain brands have high levels of certain Minerals.

Morley M. Robbins
Nexus Whole Health
1003 E. Morris Ave.
Hammond, LA 70403 USA
Email: morley@gotmag.org
(Cell: 847.922.8061)
(Skype: morleyrobbins5)

Current turnaround time is approximately 1 month, from HTMA order to HTMA consult.

You will receive a customized Excel file with your ratios, graphs and over-view, which will be used as a basis to discuss with Morley during your 60 minute consultation.

SAMPLE LETTER:
Dear Global Clients and MAG-pies!,

We're delighted that you've made the decision to assess your Mineral status through a Hair Tissue Mineral Analysis (HTMA). We're confident that you will find this testing procedure to be far more revealing about your body's state of metabolic balance, and the complete opposite of what you may have learned about it from prior conversations with friends, family, your doctor, or what may be posted about this process on the Internet.

Amount of Hair Required: 1 FULL Tbsp of hair (just enough to tip the cardboard Scale) in 1" - 1.5" lengths. Please **submit** from **4 spots** on your head, and please **discard** the rest of the hair. Experience has taught us that the best locations are above the

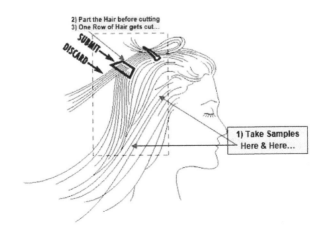

ears (Temporal Lobe) and bottom of scull in the back (Occipital Lobe) -- both left and right sides.

The hair needs to be washed within 24 hours and <u>dry</u> before sampling.

Place the hair sample in the small envelope with account # 6898, seal it, and then fill in your name and shampoo. Then, please complete the sections on the Blue Intake Form with RED *'s: Patient Demographic Info, Type of Shampoo, and Predominant Symptoms, *date it*, and then mail both to TEI Labs. Finally, please complete the Green Intake Form online, save it, and email it to the address noted below.

<u>BLUE INTAKE FORM and Hair</u>: <u>GREEN INTAKE FORM</u> :

Morley M. Robbins   **Morley M. Robbins**

Nexus Whole Health   **Email:** morley@gotmag.org

1003 E. Morris Ave.   **(Cell: 847.922.8061)**

Hammond, LA 70403 USA   (**Skype**: morleyrobbins5)

Should you be more visually inclined, please review the video link below.

http://www.youtube.com/watch?v=ze8uJO-Hs_Y

Please call or email me to clarify any questions that you might have about completing this sampling process.

morley@gotmag.org

Cheers! **Morley Robbins,** *aka "Magnesium Man!"*
You can purchase a follow up consult here:

http://gotmag.org/work-with-us/

Just select the "Health Recovery Coach" option...

Turn-around time is 7 to 10 days...

Metabolically active sources for HTMA:

o   Scalp Hair
o   Finger nails
o   Toe nails

Acceptable, but NOT nearly as active sources (they don't grow as much...)

o   Pubic hair
o   Armpit/Chest/Arm hair

And yes, Pubic hair skews the Phosphorus levels, but other minerals are very representative...

Assessing Your Mineral Status Via Bloods Tests

In a perfect world, I'd love to see:

http://requestatest.com/mag-zinc-copper-panel-testing?hc_location=ufi

o   Mag RBC
o   Plasma Zinc
o   Serum Copper
o   Serum Ceruloplasmin
o   Serum Iron
o   Serum Ferritin
o   Serum Transferrin
o   Serum TIBC (%SAT)

o   By far, virgin scalp hair is best...Absent that, here's the peaking order:
  -    Dyed, but NOT bleached (bleach or H2O2), is next... (Ideally, wait 4-6 weeks following your last dye session)
  -    Fingernails, next...
  -    Hair, south of the Border, is next..
  -    Your pets hair...and,
  -    Your best friend's scalp hair would be **last**...

Please check with your hairdresser to see what chemicals are used. When asked, "Shampoo?" please state brand and some brands contains high minerals.

Plasma Vs Serum
Because of clotting factors in Plasma vs Serum, there is intentional selection of Zinc in Plasma and Copper in Serum. There is method to this madness...

Red Blood Count Vs Serum

When we're baking cookies, it's the Oven temp that's important, NOT the Kitchen temp...

o   RBC = Oven
o   Serum = Kitchen Doctorsthe world over - hve been trained to measure the Kitchen temp, which makes no sense... Serum appears "active," but has NO bearing on our true metabolism or health status...

It's amazing actually, in March, 1961, John Kennedy gave a speech at NASA and declared we were going to the Moon! In 8 years scientists harnessed the technical know-how to get to the Moon, walk on it AND return to planet earth!

And here we are 100+ years after Karl Fiedler MD, declared that Electrolyte Derangement CAUSED disease (1899, in Vienna) -- and "scientists" are still wringing their hands "trying" to find a "valid" diagnostic tool, to measure Mg status and loss in the human...

Pleeeeeeeease, do they think we're really THAT stupid?!?...

Healthy Ranges For Blood Tests

o   Mag RBC: 5.0-7.0 mg/dL MAG goal: Strive for 6.5

o   Plasma Zinc: 100-130 mcg/dL

o   Serum Copper 80-100 mcg/dL

o   Serum Ceruloplasmin: 25-40mg/dL

o   Zinc/Usable Copper ratio: 1.3 to 1.0

o   "Usable" Copper = 3x Cp level

o   Ferritin 25-50/dL
(based on leading Cardiologist's and NOT on Thyroid Facebook Groups, lost in Iron supplementation)

Stop Supplements Before Testing

o   LabCorp has no such policy...

o   Quest says to abstain several days -- I know not why?...

This Intracellular Mg test, should be MANDATORY upon ANY doctor office visit or hospital stay. If that were the case, there would be a dramatic DECLINE in these visits...(Please, connect the dots, folks....)

Imagine the absurdity of an ER visit and being told to come back in 5 days when your system was "clear" of minerals!!!!

Who does that make sense to?!?...

I welcome anyone providing credible reasons why abstinence makes ANY sense for these essential vital mineral tests to come forward and educate us all...

Product Recommendations

When we got to this stage in the book, Morley proposed that it be discarded - at least for now. His hesitation was that he didn't want people to skip to this section, overlook the importance of having context for the symptoms that they were experiencing, and essentially "self-diagnose" with limited understanding.

It is important to know your mineral status before jumping in ANY nutrient supplementation protocol. What works for one individual, may not work for you. It is NOT a "one size fits all."

This is a brief range of a few products Morley has sourced, as he feels that they are to the highest standard.

This is a GUIDE not a diagnoses. This is a mere few recommendations, which we plan to expand over the next few books. Please remember, these companies are not affiliated with Morley, and may change their formulation at any time. If you feel there is a questionable ingredient or process, please contact Morley or the company in regards to this query.

The following recommendations have been put in here, in good faith that it is used wisely, and under the guidance of a Health Care Practitioner.

I have assured Morley, that folks who purchase these books are people who have the common sense to use these recommendations with careful consideration.

May you find what you are looking for *"A votre sante!"* - All the best, Genelle.

MTHR Natures Nutrients

Apple Cider Vinegar

Serving Size: 1 Tbsp. (15 mL)
Servings Per Container: 32
Each Serving Contains
Potassium   11mg

Blackstrap Molasses

Blackstrap molasses has very low dose of potassium, as does cream of tartar. Daily intake should be around 5000mg or more depending on your health, molasses has 1464 mg per 100gm, so that's 73.2mg per teaspoon.

What Blackstrap Molasses does for us, and for our hair - One serving (two tablespoons) of blackstrap contains approximately 14 percent of our *RDI of copper, an important trace mineral whose peptides help rebuild the skin structure that supports healthy hair. Consequently, long-term consumption of blackstrap has been linked to improved hair quality, along with the potential to encourage hair regrowth.

**Safe sweetener for diabetics - Unlike refined sugar, blackstrap molasses has a moderate glycemic load of 55. This makes it a good sugar substitute for diabetics and individuals who are seeking to avoid blood sugar spikes. Moreover, one serving of blackstrap contains no fat and only 32 calories (134 kilojoules) making it suitable for a weight loss diet when used with careful food intake. **If you should be diabetic, the use of any sugar substance should be discussed with your Medical Doctor.

Laxative qualities - blackstrap is a natural stool softener that can improve the regularity and quality of your bowel movements. Rich in iron - Two tablespoons of blackstrap contain 13.2 percent of our *RDI of iron, which our bodies need to carry oxygen to our blood cells. People who are anemic will greatly benefit from consuming 1-2 tablespoons of blackstrap molasses per day. A daily intake of blackstrap molasses can be of benefit in pregnancy, but once again, this should be discussed with your doctor.

High in calcium and magnesium - Like all whole foods, blackstrap molasses contains a mineral profile that has been optimized by nature for superior absorption. For example, two tablespoons of blackstrap contains 11.7 percent of our *RDI of calcium and 7.3 percent of our *RDI of magnesium. This calcium-magnesium ratio is ideal, since our bodies need the magnesium to help absorb the calcium. Both of these minerals aid in the growth, development and maintenance of healthy bone structure.

Additional mineral content - Two tablespoons of blackstrap molasses also contains 18 percent of our *RDI of manganese (which helps produce energy from the utilization of protein and carbohydrate), 9.7 percent of our *RDI of potassium (which plays an important role in nerve transmission and muscle contraction), 5 percent of our *RDI of vitamin B6 (which aids brain and skin development) and 3.4 percent of our *RDI of selenium, an important antioxidant.

Taking blackstrap as a health supplement The best way to take blackstrap as a supplement is to mix between 1-2 tablespoons of it in a cup of boiling water and then drink it through a straw once the water has cooled. Using a straw helps the molasses bypass your teeth. Any type of sugar coating left adhering to the teeth is not good practice. It is always beneficial for the health of your teeth and gums to clean the teeth and rinse any remaining traces of the sugar substance from the mouth.

The molasses intake ideally would be on a daily basis, and for most people, the best time is first thing in the morning.

Finally, remember to purchase only blackstrap that is organic and has not been treated with sulphur.

* Recommended daily intake.

References:-

http://www.whfoods.com

http://beforeitsnews.com

Per 2 teaspoons -

Riboflavin	.01mg	Copper	.28mg
Niacin	.15mg	Maganese	.36mg
Folate	.14mg	Selenium	2.43mcg
Vit B6	.10mg		
Calcium	117.53mg		
Iron	2.39mg		
Magnesium	29.38mg		
Phosphorus	5.47mg		
Potassium	340.57mg		
Sodium	7.52mg		
Zinc	.14mg		

Borax
(MJ Hamp's take on Borax)

A pinch in a litre of water and having one sip a day will not provide much boron.

What and How Much to Use:
In some countries (e.g. Australia, NZ, USA) borax can still be found in the laundry and cleaning sections of supermarkets. There is no "food-grade" borax available or necessary. All borax is the same and "natural", and usually mined in California or Turkey, whether it has been packed in China or any other country. The label usually states that it is 99% pure (or 990g/kg borax) which is safe to use, and is the legal standard for agricultural grade borax. Up to 1% mining and refining residues are permitted.

Boric acid, if available, may be used at about ⅔ the dose of borax, it is not for public sale in Australia.

Firstly dissolve a lightly rounded teaspoonful (5-6 grams) of borax in 1 litre of good quality water. This is your concentrated solution, keep it out of reach of small children.

Standard dose = 1 teaspoon (5 ml) of concentrate. This has 25 to 30 mg of borax and provides about 3 mg of boron. Take 1 dose per day mixed with drink or food. If that feels right then take a second dose with another meal. If there is no specific health problem or for maintenance you may continue indefinitely with 1 or 2 doses daily.

If you do have a problem, such as arthritis, osteoporosis and related conditions, cramps or spasms, stiffness due to advancing

years, menopause, and also to improve low sex hormone production, increase intake to 3 or more spaced-out standard doses for several months or longer until you feel that your problem has sufficiently improved. Then drop back to 1 or 2 doses per day.

For treating Candida, other fungi and mycoplasmas, or for removing fluoride from the body - using your bottle of concentrated solution:

Lower dose for low to normal weight - 100 ml 1/8 teaspoon of borax powder or 500 mg); drink spaced out during the day.

Higher dose for heavier individuals - 200 ml 1/4 teaspoon of borax powder or 1000 mg); drink spaced out during the day.

Always start with a lower dose and increase gradually to the intended maximum. Take the maximum amounts for 4 or 5 days a week as long as required, or reduce the maximum dose for one week each month to a minimum dose, or alternatively periodically alternate between a low dose and your maximum dose in a different rhythm.

For **vaginal thrush** fill a large size gelatine capsule with borax and insert it at bedtime for one to two weeks. With **toe fungus** or athlete's foot wet the feet and rub them with borax powder.

You may take borax mixed with food or in drinks. It is rather alkaline and in higher concentrations has a soapy taste. You may disguise this with lemon juice, vinegar or ascorbic acid.
In Europe borax and boric acid have been classified as reproductive poisons, and since December 2010 are no longer available to the public within the EU. Presently borax is still available in Switzerland (15), but shipment to Germany is not permitted. In Germany a small amount (20 - 50 grams) may be

ordered through a pharmacy as ant poison, it will be registered. Borax is presently still available from www.ebay.co.uk and can be shipped to other EU countries.

Boron tablets can be bought from health shops or the Internet, commonly with 3 mg of boron.

In some European countries, such as The Netherlands, these may still contain borax, but not in others, such as Germany, where boron is not allowed in ionic form as with borax or boric acid. While suitable as a general boron supplement, I do not know if or how well they work against Candida and mycoplasmas. Most scientific studies and individual experiences in regard to arthritis, osteoporosis, or sexual hormones and menopause were with borax or boric acid. It is not yet known if non-ionic boron is as effective as borax. To improve effectiveness I recommend 3 or more spaced-out boron tablets daily for an extended period combined with sufficient magnesium and a suitable antimicrobial program (16).
Possible Side-Effects

http://www.health-science-spirit.com/borax.htm

Liver

There are just 7 different types of animal Liver…. They all have Zn<> Cu <> Fe -- in strictly different ratios.

Grass fed Beef Liver is considered, by far, the safest and the most balanced.

I would put more emphasis on Cp production and less on booga-wooga excess Copper…

This is Affagato Allopathic residue in your thinking, which is where the true "detox" needs to occur.....
If you can't eat it try desiccated liver capsule (NOT de fatted):

www.perfectsupplements.com

The Health Benefits of Perfect Desiccated Liver
Nutrient Dense Source of High Quality Protein
Boost Energy
Boost the Immune System
Boost Metabolism
Improve Digestion
Maintain Healthy Cholesterol
Maintain Healthy Blood Sugar
Maintain Cardiovascular Health
Good Source of Naturally Occurring Copper, Zinc, and Chromium High Content of Cardio-Vascular Function Boosting CoQ10 Helps Repair DNA and RNA.

Nutritional Information for Perfect Desiccated Liver Non-Defatted Grass-Fed Beef Liver
70% Protein by Weight
2.8mg of Naturally Occurring Iron per 3g Serving (Highly bio-available Form of Iron)
969 IU of Naturally Occurring Vitamin A per 3g
Naturally Occurring Vitamin B12 per 3g Serving
High Content of All B Vitamins, including B12 Potent Source of Folic Acid

LIVER There's nothing like adding bio-available Copper –

properly balanced with Zinc & Iron -- to enhance the body's stores of this vital nutrient...

I once asked one of the world's authorities on Copper, Leslie M. Klevay, MD, PhD, what the BEST source of Copper/Zinc/Iron was? His response:

Grass-fed Beef Liver! (There was NO hesitation in his response...)

He did NOT say chicken livers, duck or goose... I checked the nutrient databases for these four forms and found that the BALANCE of the Zinc/Copper/Iron was decidedly different in BEEF than the fowl...

Maybe THAT'S why our Ancestors had Beef Liver 3-4X each month...

Size of your palm, once/week...

If it's cooked with lard, onions & garlic and NOT overcooked, it's a delicacy...

All too often, it's overcooked and becomes shoe leather...

Bottom's Up!

Nutritional Yeast

I've never heard that about the use of "fotification" of nutritional yeast... The Bragg family has a long standing and sterling reputation, and I'm not aware of any issues other than the urban myth-inspired fear that this product will cause a "yeast infection" which is, simply NOT true...

But if anyone can enlighten us to the contrary, please bring it on... I want to be confident that this centuries old practice still has value today. And as far as I know, it does...

Just make sure this is NOT coming by way of Newsmax, Livestrong, Life Extension, etc... I've lost faith in many of these sites... They are fulfilling someone else's agenda -- NOT perpetuating the truth, in my humble opinion.

I often recommend the Nutritional Yeast for a natural source of B's, and the activated form of B6 to enhance cellular uptake of Mg... Given that B's are water soluble, what doesn't get used, you lose...

Vitamin B6 + Mg-ATP = > P5P (Pyridoxine-5-Phosphate). I don't know where this process occurs, but we need - 25mgs of P5P for the average person/average "Stress!" level...

As for the Mg side, most manufacturers indicate the amount of both Chelated-Mg, as well as the "elemental-Mg" that is the portion of what is available for transaction. That amount should be 5mgs/lb body weight or 10mgs/kg...

Vitamins:

Amounts Per -	16g Serving	%DV
Thiamin	9.6mg	640%
Riboflavin	9.7mg	570%
Niacin	56.0 mg	280%
Vitamin B6	9.6 mg	480%
Folate	240 mcg	60%
Vitamin B1	27.8 mcg	130%
Pantothenic Acid	1.0 mg	10%

Minerals:

Amounts Per	16g Serving	%DV
Iron	0.7mg	4%

Magnesium	24.0mg	6%
Sodium	5.0mg	0%
Zinc	3.0mg	20%
Copper	0.1mg	6%
Manganese	0.1mg	6%

Read More

http://nutritiondata.self.com/facts/custom/1323565/2#ixzz3WsVpz8QP

Olive Oil

Olive Oil is your friend to elevate Cholesterol, naturally...

The connection is that:

o Low Copper >> High Cholesterol...

o Low Manganese >> Low Cholesterol...

 Olive Oil is rich in Mn...

Adrenal Support

We regularly use this form from Medi-Herb, but it is only through practitioners:

http://www.standardprocess.com/Product/MediHerb/Ashwaganda-11#.Vkq6mxuooxg

This looks to be a good alternative also:

http://organicindiausa.com/organic-india-ashwagandha/?gclid+CNmKnsyh_clCFa5AMgodahMA1W

Australia Medi- Herb Supplier -

http://www.naturopathvitamins.com.au/index.php/test-menu-shop

Improve Respiratory Strength

Anderson's Sea Minerals...

My partner, Dr. Liz, starts the nutritional response testing with a bottle of Anderson's Sea MD.... I don't think there hasn't been a client who's neurological "lock" didn't get notably STRONGER with this mineral source in their energy field....

Aussie Sea Minerals

http://www.mmsaustralia.com.au/index.php?act=viewProd&productId=29

Serving size 5 ml (1 teaspoon, start with 5 drops and build): Ocean Derived Sea Minerals.

Contains 108 minerals, some of them are:

Sodium 90mg,
Potassium 116mg,
Calcium 0.2mg,
Magnesium 422mg,
Sulphur 69mg,
Carbon 109mg.................
250 mls (50 days supply)

Cod Liver Oil

o   Rosita's Extra Virgin CLO

Nordic Naturals has TWO versions:

o   Arctic: for those seeking CLO like their great-
       grandparents...

o   Arctic-D: for seeking NOT to see their grand-children...

Please note, it is the ratio of Vit-A to Vit-D that makes this
product appealing, as is its processing procedure.

Retinol, animal-based Vit-A, is your best bet. (It takes 12 Beta
Carotene & Zinc to equal 1 Retinol)

Beef liver & Cod Liver Oil are your richest sources. Some folks
prefer desiccated tablets, but I'm assuming the potency drops, in
those products due to processing... Ideally, focus on foods that
will deliver all the fat soluble vitamins (A, D, E, & K)

Supplement Facts			
Serving Size: 1 Teaspoon (5 ml)			
Servings Per Bottle: 48			
	Amount Per Serving	% DV¹	% DV²ᵃ
Calories	45		
Calories from fat	45		
Total Fat	5.0 g	†	8%
Saturated Fat	1.0 g	†	5%
Trans Fat	0 g	†	†
Cholesterol	20 mg	†	7%
Vitamin A	425-1500 I.U.	17-60%	9-30%
Vitamin D	0-20 I.U.	0-5%	0-5%
Total Omega-3s	1050 mg	†	†
EPA (Eicosapentaenoic Acid)	350 mg	†	†
DHA (Docosahexaenoic Acid)	485 mg	†	†
Other Omega-3s	215 mg	†	†

* Percent Daily Values are based on a 2,000 calorie diet.
† Daily Value not established.
¹ Daily Value (DV) for children under 4 years of age
² Daily Value (DV) for adults and children over 4 years of age

I believe your ancient ancestors INVENTED Cod Liver Oil....

WHY?

Because they knew that animal-based supplements provided ALL the nutrients & cofactors AND in the correct BALANCE.

Hormone-D MUST be balanced with 10-25X MORE retinol so that the body STAYS IN BALANCE...

Health is about Homeostasis -- NOT taking one over hyped nutrient at the expense of its biological partners in the body.

If 6 pills contain 1000IU in total of Vit-D

That level of Hormone-D needs to be matched with ~10,000 IUs of Retinol (animal-based Vit-A, NOT beta carotene, by the way...).

In my humble opinion, Carlson's is NOT a properly balanced blend... it is 2X Vit-A to 1X Vit-D...

In contrast, Nordic Naturals - Arctic is 10X Vit-A to 1X Vit-D -- THAT'S the scale of contrast needed...

When there is TOO MUCH Hormone-D, Vit-A CAN NOT do its job(s)... despite its lower cost, and it's greater popularity... Our metabolism doesn't give a lick about either one...

If you don't you run the risk of intensifying your load of bio-UN-available Copper as the lack of Vit-A will prevent production of Ceruloplasmin (Cp), which is ESSENTIAL for Copper metabolism...

Epsom Salts

Epsom salt, named for a bitter saline spring at Epsom in Surrey, England, is not actually salt but a naturally occurring pure mineral compound of magnesium and Sulfate. Long known as a natural remedy for a number of ailments. Epsom Salt has numerous health benefits within the body, including regulating the activity of enzymes, reducing inflammation, helping muscle and nerve function and helping to prevent artery hardening. Sulfates help improve the absorption of nutrients, flush toxins and help ease migraine headaches.

I would also remind you that we ARE living "1984!" where Black is white & White is black...

Examples:

o	Articles "D"emonize Epsom Salts but tell how "good" Fluoride is in our water...

o	Articles "D"emonize "grass fed" butter, yet tell us the "benefits" of GMO-laden Soy & Canola oil...

o	Articles "D"emonize Vit-A as "toxic," but glorify the use of Hormone-D...

It is ALL Affagato... It's very frustrating, but that's the world we live in now... We must challenge & question EVERYTHING that's being pumped out of Main Stream Media (whether Media or Medicine)!

Is it dangerous to take 100mg of B6 daily?
That level of B6 would likely be a good max to shoot for, but I'd ease there & not jump to that level…

Gymnema Supports Sugar Cravings

http://www.mediherb.com/product_pdf/GymnemaLR.pdf

https://www.standardprocess.com/Products/MediHerb/Gymnema#.Vsdsvgccsuk

Jigsaw Magnesium -

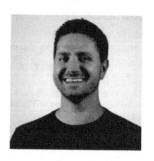

http://www.jigsawhealth.com/

Represented by Patrick Sullivan Jr. -
Founding MAG member and one of
Morley's Mentors. This is the product
Morley has personally used for the past
four years.

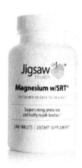

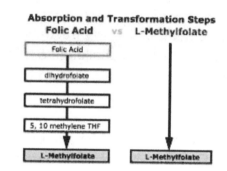

Absorption and Transformation Steps
Folic Acid   vs   L-Methylfolate

Folic Acid

dihydrofolate

tetrahydrofolate

5, 10 methylene THF

L-Methylfolate   L-Methylfolate

What about its Folic Acid??

It's NOT "Folic Acid..." I believe the term is "quadromethylfolate"
Ask the FDA why "Folic Acid" must be used when it's not in the
product...

Liver Support

Many dynamics and imbalances can affect Liver function...

o   Milk Thistle… as a herbal tonic..

Australian Stockist -

http://www.naturopathvitamins.com.au/index.php/test-menu-shop/product/34-mediherb-silymarin-milk-thistle-or-st-marys-thistle-60-tablets

o   Standard Process Livaplex… and maybe Hepatrophin
         PMG (it might also be advisable to do their 21-day
         Cleanse)

https://www.standardprocess.com/Products/Standard-Process/Hepatrophin-PMG#.Vsh59gccsul

https://www.standardprocess.com/Products/Standard-Process/Livaplex#.Vsh6p2ccsuk

o   BioRay Liver Life
http://www.bioray.com/liver-life/

Those are three very different approaches but are proven
products to restore balance and function to a Liver in need…..

MolyCu

http://www.wellnessshoppingonline.com/endo-met-supplements/moly-cu-180-tabs/

ReMag

ReMag has been legendary in its ability to help folks with Mg
issues. I'm not as well-versed on Re-Lyte to address Copper
issues, largely because resolving Copper REQUIRES resolving
Ceruloplasmin production that has been the target of dysfunction
for decades & we were ALL in the "D"ark re that... You might also
look into http://www.wateroz.com/ for their Cu water…

Products to help Yeast/Candida Infection

o   Probiotics are a good way to offset Yeast...
o   Wholefood Vit-C
o   Turpentine on a sugar cube (I kid you not...)
o   Bee Pollen...
o   Goat Yoghurt...
o   Goose Liver pate...
Those are all rich sources of Copper...

It needs to be ultra-distilled Turpentine: Diamand G Forest
Products in Georgia, USA is one distributor...

http://diamondgforestproducts.net/shop/32-oz-100-pure-gum-spirits-of-turpentine/

Wholefood Vitamin C Complex

The vast majority of "Vit-C" sold and used in America/ the World
is actually Ascorbic Acid, which is only 1/6th of the Vitamin that
Albert Zvent-Gyorgi. PhD won the Nobel Prize for.

What you need is wholefood Vit-C COMPLEX"
o   Innate Response (tablets, NOT powder)
o   Grown By Nature
o   Garden of Life
o   Mega Foods
o   Standard Process (Cataplex C)
o   Pure Synergy - Pure Radiance - Organic Berries
o   Health Force Naturals - Truly Natural Vitamin C (powder)

Yes, it makes a world of difference INSIDE your body and
INSIDE your cells.....

Whole food C products - Berries ETC I'm encouraging folks to CHECK with the manufacturers to see:

o   How much wholefood Vit-C?...

o   How much Ascorbic Acid?...

If the company cannot or will not tell you -- then that's NOT a product you need. The ones devoted to natural wholefood Vit-C will be delighted to tell you how much you're getting...

SELECTED BOOK REFERENCES

Among Morley's Favorites:

o   Carolyn Dean's "The Magnesium Miracle"

o   Robert G. Thompson's "The Calcium Lie I and II"

o   Andrea Rosanoff/Mildred Seelig, "The Magnesium Factor"

o   Rick Malter's, "The Strands of Health"

o   Carl C. Pfeiffer's, "Mental & Elemental Nutrients"

o   Gary Taubes', "Good Calories, Bad Calories"
    Gary Taubes', "Why We Get Fat"

o   Davis Kessler's, "The End Of Overeating"

o   Michael Pollan's, The Omnivore's Dilemma" and "Food Rules"

o   Byron Richards', "Fight For Your Health"

o   Weston A. Price's, "Nutrition and Physical Degeneration"

o   Byron J Richard's, "Mastering Leptin"

o   David L Watts, DC, PhD's "Trace Elements and Other Essential Nutrients."

o   Cate Shyamalan, MD's, "Deep Nutrition."

o   Sean Croxton's, The Dark Side Of Fat Loss"

No order of preference.

Morley's Favorite Facebook Sites:
Regarding Minerals

Magnesium Advocacy Group

https://www.facebook.com/groups/MagnesiumAdvocacy/

Copper Dysregulation and Re-balancing

https://www.facebook.com/groups/347066448791517/

Mag~nificent Mommies

https://www.facebook.com/groups/716503481736105/

Mineral Power Support

https://www.facebook.com/groups/mineralpower/

Concluding Thoughts From Morley

"The process of writing uncovers our own deepest thoughts and emotions then transforms them into a medium of teaching for others."
~ Harold Klemp ~

It is somewhat humbling to reach this point in this process... the "Conclusion" – at least for Vol II!

I know for a fact, that there are other volumes of these *Musings from MAG* that are in the developmental stage, and other books planned beyond that. But, it is time for a respite from this set of reflections.

Musings is not your typical "book" and its creation is the shared collaboration of yours truly and Genelle Young, who graciously volunteered to put this set of Facebook threads together, without my knowledge, and sent it to me with an innocent question: "So, what do you think?..." The irony is that MJ Hamp, the Administrator for MAG, had undertaken that very same approach – almost two years previously. However, I was just getting my Facebook legs at the time, and was not aware of what the "potential for publishing" these daily comments and reflections were from the MAG site.

I'm walking much better, now, and I'm decidedly more awake...

It is my fervent hope that you are, as well, having gotten to this point of this document.

This book lacks the traditional trappings of most published works. It is an organic and verbatim reflection of commentary provided on the MAG website. It lacks footnotes, indexes and a story line that is typically found in the world of conventional publishing. The approach we are electing to take is one of expediency: to make these insights and observations about mineral nutrition, and its impact upon our metabolism, available to a much broader audience, given that many, many MAG-pies seem to have found them beneficial and supportive to their efforts to heal and attain mineral balance and improved well being.

But, unlike traditional books, it will have the benefit of updates and added insights as they evolve and are warranted with new information.

As I sit back and reflect on what I want you to walk away with having finished reading this document, I truly want you to do the following:

- o ***Question more....***
  The REAL purpose of this book is not so much to beat my chest about what I know, but give you a very different context for the knowledge that you think you know. This book's ultimate intention is to grant you the strength of conviction to challenge what you know, and challenge those traditional sources of information. Ask more questions... do more research... exercise your critical thinking skills wherever possible – but certainly as it relates to your mineral nutrition and your health.

- o ***Believe more...***
  Especially believe more in the innate capacity of your body to heal itself. Our body is designed to reach homeostasis... to get back to an even keel. Know that, and have faith in restorative powers of your body and your mind. But there is one pre-requisite: feed the body REAL food and wherever

possible, wholefood supplements. That's where the "genuine replacement parts" are for the billion cells you lose each and every hour due to the natural cycle of cell death and cell replacement. Know that your innate healer is there to serve you... it just needs to be nourished, especially with minerals. – the spark plugs of life!

o ***Share more...***
My wildest dream is that each member of MAG will buy at least 10 copies of this book. Not because of the opportunity to make some money (although my creditors would actually like THAT for a change...), but far more importantly that this metabolic <u>truth</u> about minerals become a household phrase and way of life, that we end this tyranny of "mother may I" with mainstream medicine. I, for one, am done with that, have pledged my remaining days on this Planet to spreading that truth regularly, repeatedly, and rightfully. It's time for a much larger percentage of our world population to know these truths, as well.

o ***Express gratitude more...***
Among the many things that I've learned over the last several years of doing wellness and HTMA consults is that when we're feeling ill, uncomfortable, or out of sync with our norm, we ALL have a tendency to find fault, express frustration and think about what we DON'T have. And how does the Universe *always* respond? By taking away EVEN MORE... So, it's time we all take stock of how to STOP that. All we need do is express heartfelt gratitude for the many, many blessings that grace our lives. And even when we're feeling our worst, there is STILL much to be thankful for. And when we engage in that regular

practice of expressing our heartfelt gratitude, despite our pains and discomfort, how does the Universe *always* respond? By giving us MORE. It never fails and that disciplined act ALSO activates the Parasympathetic Nervous System which is the side if ANS, command & control center for Rest & Recovery... the very part of our healing factors that is so often overlooked. Please, just say "Thank you!" more.

o ***Gain independence more...***
At the heart of this entire effort of educating folks about minerals, and Maggie, and her Yin/Yang partner, Copper, is the expressed intention that we ALL reach a state of health independence that frees us from worry, fear, doubt, frustration and allows us to attain our TRUE purpose in this lifetime. I can assure you, we were NOT meant to suffer endlessly or stay trapped inside bodies and minds that are either NOT balanced, NOR behaving properly or fully. The more we focus on the mineral foundation that runs our body, the more we can take control of the metabolism that, in fact, runs our bodies. Again, as I've noted elsewhere in the book, there is no such thing as medical disease... there is ONLY metabolic dysfunction that is CAUSED by mineral deficiencies... That is my favorite belief and the basis of my approach to wellness coaching.

So, I will close with those thoughts.

Thank you for your time and attention. I very much appreciate the investment you have made to get to this point in the book. I also want you to know that I welcome your questions and comments about what you've read. Start a thread on MAG, drop me an email, or pick up the phone – Please know, I've NEVER met a question that I didn't enjoy. So I look forward to the feedback and the opportunity to refine this message, and address others that you, the reader, and those in you circle of family and friends, feel warrant.

Made in the USA
Middletown, DE
02 March 2024

50667827R00176